DYSLEXIA
AND ADHD—
THE MIRACLE CURE

WYNFORD DORE
WITH DAVID BROOKES

JOHN BLAKE

Published by John Blake Publishing Ltd,
3 Bramber Court, 2 Bramber Road,
London W14 9PB, England

www.johnblakepublishing.co.uk

www.facebook.com/Johnblakepub facebook
twitter.com/johnblakepub twitter

First published in paperback in 2008
This edition published in paperback in 2013

ISBN: 978 185782 688 3

British Library Cataloguing-in-Publication Data:

A catalogue record for this book is available from the British Library.

Design by www.envydesign.co.uk

Printed and bound in Great Britain by CPI Group (UK) Ltd

1 3 5 7 9 10 8 6 4 2

Papers used by John Blake Publishing are natural, recyclable products made
from wood grown in sustainable forests. The manufacturing processes conform to
the environmental regulations of the country of origin.

Every attempt has been made to contact the relevant copyright-holders, but some
were unobtainable. We would be grateful if the appropriate people could contact us.

CONTENTS

ACKNOWLEDGEMENTS

I am just one piece of a smallish organisation tackling a huge problem worthy of a really large institute. It should have been Harvard Medical School, Oxford University or some highly resourced organisation pursuing this. Research from these wonderful establishments has been vital of course but piecing it all together has only happened because of the passionate commitment and contribution of each and every one of a number of folk working with me in the team, and these I have to thank. There is not space to include everyone but I will mention some.

First, Susie – she had the desperate need, she had obvious hidden abilities and thus provided the inspiration. To Mum – for instilling in me that life is good when you are helping others who need it. My partner Julie, who kept me sane and alive. Roy Rutherford for piecing the medical research together (and being the only doctor mad enough to listen); Evelyn – the best secretary in the world; Professors Nicolson and Reynolds; Professors Schmahmann and Price. Dr Ned Hallowell, Trevor Davies, Bob

Brolly, Carolyn, Rachel, Ian, Joe, Tim, John, Susan, Susanne, Polly, Pam, Rosie, Peter Morley, Kenny, Toyah, Julie, John McDermott and every other member of our team and all the families that gave it a go so we could conduct our research. I count myself very lucky to have Phil Hall as a friend and adviser, to have David Brookes who made the task of putting this together so much easier and a wonderful publisher who realised the need to share this breakthrough with everyone. What a crew!

FOREWORD

ar too many people are still needlessly struggling with reading, struggling with attention issues, struggling with co-ordination and, if all that wasn't bad enough, often struggling with poor short-term memory as well. Research is showing that 80% of those with reading difficulties also have attention difficulties and, in an attempt to address this, we have changed the title for this paperback edition to include reference to 'ADHD'. Research suggests that the root cause of all of these symptoms lies in one part of the cerebellar, and that by developing that one area, many (if not all), of those symptoms improve significantly. This is why it is so important to address the source of these symptoms.

The approach described in this book is not a 'one size fits all' approach; it's an individualised approach that focuses on bringing out all of the hidden potential of that individual. One surprising aspect of the results we see is that, often, a large number of further skills are improved over the course of the programme. This is in contrast to the many interventions that

tackle these problems from the symptom end – there are usually too many symptoms to be able to deal with them all individually, hence tackling the root cause is a far better idea altogether.

It was expected that the hardback edition of this book would be controversial, and it was. Thousands seemed to appreciate 'an explanation at last' and then there were a few who didn't like it so much. Most of this latter group fitted into two categories; they were either specialists in phonics or they are engaged in research funded directly or indirectly by drug companies. So the arguments continue to abound 'Does dyslexia exist?', 'Can it be cured?' or 'Is ADHD just an excuse?' If we just asked teachers and parents these same questions we could get some very clear answers. By then asking them 'What works?' we would get some more enlightening answers.

This paperback edition is being prepared at a time when yet another research study on reading has just been published. This latest study says that the British Government has spent half a billion pounds in the last few years on literacy interventions with no real impact on reading ability. What a disappointment (but maybe no surprise) to those who are suffering, all their families and all those teachers who put their heart, mind and soul into taking the latest advice from education advisors about how to teach those with dyslexic type symptoms. This book shows that these failures are not the fault of teachers or parents. An international benchmarking standard is desperately needed for all educational interventions. Only when that has happened will we be able to determine the best and most effective tools to use in our classrooms.

A recent and important development for all educational professionals and parents is the availability of an on-line assessment (ACE) that is neurologically based, fun for kids to do and provides teachers and parents with vital data about the

underlying potential that a child may have. How amazing will a teacher find it to run a simple computer-based assessment on all pupils in the class to get an understanding of their learning style, to ascertain who has hidden potential and who in the class is working exceptionally hard to achieve their results? When it is used more generally it will make us focus on the enormous talent that so many children have despite their being constrained by the physiological reasons that makes reading or concentrating for long periods difficult.

And there is more hope – a US-based charity is funding a very large independent study on the effect of the theories behind the Dore Programme. It is hoped that it will not only provide crucial data on the various symptoms being addressed but may also provide a blueprint for benchmarking that can be applied to all interventions used for these symptoms.

INTRODUCTION

A Miracle Cure? was the title of a major documentary programme produced in the UK and shown on ITV's *Tonight with Trevor McDonald*. The programme took an unprecedented, detailed look at the work Dore Achievement Centre had done in tackling learning difficulties. It triggered record-breaking interest in two different and surprising ways.

First, there were hundreds of thousands of attempts to phone our offices, made by people whose lives were being blighted by the symptoms they had witnessed during the documentary. These included poor reading skills, poor writing ability, poor concentration and often a low self-esteem. Some had even been called stupid or lazy, which is particularly cruel as we have now discovered that usually these folk are potentially brighter and are working harder than others. They had watched the show and marvelled as people with these problems had been transformed, and they wanted to find out how they could have this groundbreaking treatment themselves.

Most of them had not had those symptoms diagnosed, although some had been labelled as suffering from ADHD

(Attention Deficit Hyperactivity Disorder), dyslexia, dyspraxia or, in a few cases, Asperger's Syndrome. As a consequence of that television programme, many of those people have now had their lives totally transformed.

The second response to the documentary was from the learning difficulties industry offended by the documentary maker's claims of 'a revolutionary breakthrough' in the treatment of dyslexia and the possibility of a cure. When used, cure is a word that seems to cause great offence to many professionals and for this reason we have always chosen to avoid using it. But the fact is the drug-free exercise-based programme we have developed is now delivering amazing results, and research says that the results seem permanent – the question is as to how best those results are described. Is 'cure' the best word to use?

Families that have to live with the symptoms of learning difficulties every day would love to have a solution for them, but up until now they may not have been aware that one may exist. Why is that? Well, most of those with symptoms of learning difficulties are brighter than average – behind that mask of symptoms that is. But, because the underlying cause of these problems has been misunderstood, virtually all treatments or programmes developed to deal with them up until now have had only mediocre impact. Thus, our life-changing programme presented quite a threat to that industry.

The fact is we are not a threat. There are two aspects to the process of learning – the first is a physiological one; the brain must have the ability to learn – that is what we work on. The other aspect is the process of 'teaching', and of course that is what teachers (and parents) do every day. For learning to be possible, both are needed. So, what we are doing is repairing the hole in the bucket; teaching is filling that bucket.

I am writing this at a time when it has just been announced in the US that many prescription drugs provided to treat ADHD sufferers must now have a black box on their label, warning of potential harmful side-effects. So it will be a great relief to families to know that the effectiveness of this exercise programme on ADHD is quite remarkable. Research has shown it to have twice the effectiveness of drugs, with no side-effects and when it is complete – typically after a year – it is permanent. How much better to spend five minutes twice a day for a few months to have a long-term solution not just to attention and hyperactivity issues but to unlocking the patient's underlying potential, too. There's no contest!

Of course, sadly, there are some who have very complex needs that the methods described in this book can't always help. However, a startling one in six of the population is hampered by conditions we believe can be helped, and with the size of the problem it will ultimately require the resources of governments so that it reaches everyone who needs it.

But how long will this take? And will those with vested interests make sure its impact will be held up with the consequence that another generation will needlessly suffer? Will this paradigm shift take as long to be brought into use as penicillin did, for example, before it is accepted? And was Trevor McDonald's right to raise the suggestion that this might, in time, lead to a cure?

The fact is, the results are amazing and, while what we share with you is still a theory, the science behind the outcomes is increasingly well understood. The need, too, is a desperate one and personally I care less about which word is used. Instead, I will focus all my energies on getting this wonderful hope and help to those who need it, fast.

CONTACT INFORMATION
FOR SCREENING TESTS AND OTHER
RESEARCH INFORMATION

wynforddore@hotmail.co.uk

Chapter 1

SUSIE'S STORY — MY DAUGHTER WITH DYSLEXIA AND ADHD

(ATTENTION DEFICIT HYPERACTIVITY DISORDER)

Surely, there is no worse feeling in the world than having your child tell you that she does not want to go on living. As I stood by my 25-year-old daughter's bedside in hospital, where she was recovering from her third suicide attempt, I remember feeling utterly helpless. I felt lonely, desperate and useless. I also felt anger towards the Establishment for not having the answer to her problem.

Like so many parents in the world, I had a child who suffered from a learning problem. Looking back, my greatest regret is my lack of understanding of the condition when she was growing up. At the time, I just could not believe that something could go into a person's head and not stay there. I had never experienced that myself and my other children picked things up with great ease. Because I could not understand her problem, I was not there for Susie in the way she needed me to be. Now I realise how she felt, I will never get over the guilt.

At this point, it must be stated that the problems that Susie

had were considerably more severe than many of the people who were to go through the programme we have developed. Most of the people we have helped over the last few years have displayed considerably milder symptoms than the ones Susie had. The reason I want to make this point clear is that it would be a great shame for parents to read my daughter's story and assume that, because their child may not be affected by learning or attention difficulties as severely as she was, this programme is not for them. Indeed, Susie is an extreme example of the type of person who comes to us. Nevertheless, if it had not been for her, the whole programme would never have existed.

LIVING WITH A LEARNING OR ATTENTION PROBLEM

The more I come to understand about what Susie was going through, the more I look back in anguish at how she must have felt. For her, each day was a nightmare. When she got up in the morning all she could think about was the prospect of going to school and how she felt different and inferior to the others around her. In her lessons, she would constantly make all kinds of mistakes. She seemed to be unable to grasp simple concepts, learn from them and mentally develop like the other students.

If she ever did manage to learn anything one day, by the next morning it would have vaporised from her mind, and she would be back to square one. I remember clearly trying to teach Susie simple three- and four-letter words, and she would just look back at me with a blank expression; she could not take it in. It was as if something was wrong with the wiring in her head, stopping her from retaining anything. One day, we spent hours going over her four times table until eventually she seemed to have got it. However, the next morning at breakfast, I gave her a little test and she did not have a clue.

2

I used to feel extremely frustrated, but also very puzzled about her seeming inability to learn. In some circumstances, she was able to run rings around me. I could see she had a creative mind, which showed itself in all sorts of ways. For example, she would often say something highly intelligent, which would surprise me to the core. However, the next day if I asked her about it, she would not be able to remember what she had said. It was almost as if she had found a way to manipulate her own IQ, as if she could turn it on – or off – at will.

Of course, I now know that this was not the case. Just as I was frustrated and did not know what was going on, so was Susie equally frustrated and confused. The difference was that she had to live with that frustration. Although I was really worried about her, at least I could have a respite. I could go to my job and escape from it. She had to deal with the fact that schoolwork was impossible, organising herself was impossible, completing any task was impossible. She was not simply failing academically; in social situations, she also faced huge obstacles.

When Susie was growing up, she had communication problems. This was largely down to the fact her verbal processing speed was much slower than it should have been. Often what she wanted to say would just not come to her mind quickly enough and so the conversation would move on before she had time to contribute. This meant that girls of her age could not relate to her and while growing up she had few friends. As other children learned more and more, and grew in social awareness, Susie barely moved forward at all. Most of her friends were either much older than she was, or much younger. With these friends, she felt that she did not have to struggle so much; she could just concentrate on having fun and not worry about showing herself up.

3

She seemed to have absolutely no concept of the consequences of her actions, which caused much grief and frustration to those around her. She simply did not know how to ask for things. When she wanted something, she would just go ahead and take it. This caused all sorts of problems with her siblings, as, for instance, she would go into their room, take their music tapes without asking permission and not put them back.

Even the simplest of tasks would become a huge chore for her. I remember how I would give her £10 and ask her to go to the local newsagents to buy a newspaper. Hours later, she would return with the wrong newspaper and no change. In frustration, I would sometimes shout at her for being careless. This would, of course, always result in tears and she would run to her bedroom and slam the door.

Looking back, I now know that she was not being deliberately careless at all. She simply couldn't help being unstructured and disorganised in her everyday life; she had no alternative. At the time, none of us understood this and Susie was constantly in trouble. Because of her poor verbal processing, she was also the butt of many of her siblings' jokes. While we, as parents, did all that we could to contain this, children will always be children and I am quite sure such ribbing happened constantly behind our backs.

No doubt, this contributed to the desperate feeling of loneliness Susie had to endure for the whole of her childhood. I remember the day of her fifteenth birthday and we invited a number of children around. Of course, most of these children were Rosie and Glyn's friends because Susie did not find it as easy to make friends. This meant that everyone was playing with her brother and sister, and she was ignored even though it was her birthday. She was not involved in the game of cricket, she was not

involved in the after-tea card games and she spent most of the time lost in her own world because her verbal processing was so slow she simply couldn't comfortably relate to others.

Because of her learning problems, we sent Susie to a private school. This was because I felt that in a state school, where there can often be over 30 pupils in one class, there was no way a teacher, despite their best efforts, would be able to give her the attention she needed. She went to a small school called Abbotsford School in Kenilworth, Warwickshire. As I did not want Susie to feel different to my other children, I ended up sending all my kids to the same school.

When Susie was nine years old, her teacher came to me and told me she thought she was dyslexic. Thank goodness that teacher had the astuteness to point out to me what was then a rarely recognised condition. As a consequence, we took her to see Dr Margaret Newton, a psychologist specialising in dyslexia and formerly of Aston University in Birmingham, who confirmed that Susie did indeed have dyslexia. I remember the whole way through the meeting Susie was restless and could not sit still. She spent much of the time looking out of the window and avoiding eye contact with anyone in the room. By this point, she really was just tagging along in life. She was unable to understand major concepts like dyslexia and she would much rather have been in her room, passively watching the world drift by.

Abbotsford was a wonderful little school that had a track record of getting children through their entrance exams to senior schools in the area. The teachers were some of the most intelligent and caring people I have ever met and were committed to helping Susie get over her problems. Despite this, she went right through her education retaining very little. The school, of course, was aware of her problem and needed to put her in classes with

younger children. This was terribly embarrassing for her and she still recalls being 12 years old and sitting in a class with eight-year-olds, learning how to spell three- or four-letter words.

For a long time, Susie worked very hard. However, as you can imagine, she made very little headway. I remember dreading parents' evenings. Susie's mother and I would always have to take a deep breath before sitting down to talk to one of her teachers. We knew it would not be good news, we knew it would be difficult to take in. It was particularly hard because her two younger siblings Rosie and Glyn were flying academically and getting glowing reports. I remember coming home one evening from parents' evening to find Rosie and Glyn waiting for us at the door. They were all excited, positive and upbeat, and wanted to know what had been said about them. In direct contrast, Susie was sitting in the corner of the room, with her head down and headphones on. She was too scared and embarrassed to ask us how it went; she knew what the answer would be.

I found myself repeatedly telling her off for making the same mistakes. As a parent, I felt that I had to do this because it was my only tool to try to get her to focus. In absolute honesty, I was at my wits' end and I did not know what else to do with her. I had sent her to the best school in the area and she had met with the top research experts. Yet still she was not making progress. I could not think of anything else I could do – if I could have, I would have done it. Susie had gone to the Dyslexia Institute in Coventry in her early teens and tried their methods but to no avail. Indeed, we had tried all the teaching and reading programmes the experts could throw at us but nothing seemed to work.

Despite all the things I had done in my business life, I felt like a complete failure. Susie was desperately lonely and I could not do anything. I was helpless and hopeless. Although I loved my

daughter and I wanted her to be happy, by this point even I accepted there was no way forward. I had not given up on her, but I felt that it was ultimately up to her to come to terms with the problem. It is no wonder then that she became withdrawn, choosing to spend more time on her own in her bedroom. Music and television became her best friends and she shunned the outside world. She used to come home from school and eat dinner with the family. As soon as she had finished her meal, she would run upstairs, into her bedroom, where she would remain until the next day.

> 'Meal times were particularly difficult for me. I was not allowed to wear my Walkman so I'd have to listen to the others gabbling on. I couldn't keep up with what they were saying and if I wanted to say something I just couldn't find the words until it was too late. By the end of the meal, I was just desperate to get away so I could bury my head in my pillow and cry. I would cry so much that I would have to turn my pillow over because it would get so wet.
>
> 'Things were so much better in my room. I could listen to my music and watch the soap operas that I loved. I did not have a life with my own family, or with my school that was worth living. All I remember from those times is a black loneliness. I did not want to be alive.'

The hardest thing was when Susie used to ask me, 'Why am I different? Why is it that other kids are picked first for teams but I am left for last?' But I would never have an appropriate answer. I would want to cry and tell her, 'I do not know why you cannot learn! I do not know why your brother and sisters can grasp things straight away, but you need to be told again and again.'

The difficulty of helping Susie was compounded by the fact that she did not seem to want any help. Every time that we, her family, tried to support her, Susie would push us away and retreat inside her room and inside herself. She did not want our sympathy. Behind the façade of a weak and socially inept person was a strong, independently minded woman who wanted to be self-empowered and independent. She did not want to feel that she had to rely on her family to be happy. Sometimes, I felt like the best way to help her was not to help her at all, hoping that time would be her cure.

I hoped that as her teenage years faded behind her and she became an adult she would develop coping strategies so that, little by little, her self-confidence would build up and she would one day feel 'normal'. Tragically, Susie slipped further and further into a depressed state. She imprisoned herself away from the world and eventually tried to take her own life. This experience taught me in the most painful way possible the grief that many parents around the world face every day.

MY DAUGHTER TRIES TO KILL HERSELF

I will never forget the feeling of absolute despair when I received a phone call from Rosie to say my daughter had tried to kill herself. Although I was aware that she had been depressed, I had not realised just how bad things had become for her. I also failed to make the direct connection between her learning and attention difficulties and her unsettled state of mind. When, as a family, we talked about her depression, we discussed it as if it were virtually a stand-alone issue. We never imagined that the root cause of all of her school problems could be directly linked to her depression.

Of course, with the benefit of hindsight, it is all so painfully obvious. We now know that what causes learning difficulties can

have a detrimental effect on so many characteristics. For instance, nearly 90 per cent of folk who attempt to commit suicide show signs typical of learning or attention issues and as many as 75 per cent of people who have long-term drug addictions have signs of similar issues too.

For Susie, her decline and attempt to take her own life had been years in the making. Every attempt to learn, to develop friendships or to hold down a job had resulted in failure. It did not matter how much her family had tried to help her, life would never cease to be a struggle.

I had bought an apartment for her in Leamington Spa when she was 19, as she really wanted to live by herself and she and I both thought this would help her become more comfortable with the problems she faced. However, that only made things worse. Sitting in her flat by herself she says she would hear my voice in her head saying things like 'Why can't you get a job? Why can't you stick at something useful? Why can't you do this? Why can't you do that?' She would then start crying, but instead of getting angry with me she would mentally beat herself up for hours on end.

The mistake we made was to assume Susie had a choice in her actions. We told her she would have to learn to hold down a job, to learn to get on with people. We thought many of her failures in life came down to the fact that she could not be bothered to make an effort. Unwittingly, what we were telling her to do was the exact thing she could never achieve: she could not learn – it was not an option. The more we told her how she needed to behave, the further she retreated into herself.

Things quickly got out of hand and in a four-year period, during the mid-nineties, Susie had tried to kill herself three times.

The first incident (when she was 22 years old), as she now

freely admits, was perhaps more a cry for help than a serious attempt at suicide. However, the message she was sending out was clear and calculated. By her bedside, she had written many little notes obviously intended for me to read. They read like a series of short, sharp statements designed to cut me deeper than the knife had cut her arm:

'My life is terrible!' 'I hate myself!' 'Why are you always shouting at me?'

These were thoughts that had dominated her life but she had always struggled to express them. All around her people were getting on with their lives and she felt more and more left behind. Her decision to cut her wrists was an act of defiance at the way her life was going. It put her whole family in a state of absolute panic and anxiety.

By the time of the second attempt, Susie was 23 years old and was living by herself with hardly any quality of life at all. She was not eating properly and spent most of her time curled up on the sofa watching TV and drinking wine. On one particularly soul-destroying and lonely night, she decided enough was enough and, after consuming three bottles of wine, she rounded up as many pills as she could lay her hands on. Before she had a chance to do anything, the phone rang – it was her mother calling to check how she was.

Susie recalls wanting to tell her mum how depressed she was, but she couldn't find the words. As soon as she put down the phone, she resumed the task she had set herself. She took a handful of about six headache tablets and had another bottle of wine. It was no small mercy that this had the effect of knocking her out so that she did not take any more harmful pills that night.

In the morning, she woke up with a splitting headache and in a state of severe depression. She spent the day wandering

aimlessly about the house and in the end decided to keep the details of her suicide attempt a secret. It was not until her third and final attempt that we ever found out how close we had come to losing her on that night.

Things became progressively worse and Susie got to the stage where she could barely look after herself, let alone function as a social human being. Every day her mother and sister would phone her to make sure she had got out of bed and to check that she had eaten her breakfast. They would ask her about her plans for the day and try to motivate her as much as they could. Despite all their best efforts, Susie continued to fall deeper and deeper into depression. She felt patronised and was tired of being treated like a child. Of course, we were aware of this, but it seemed there was nothing else any of us could do. We knew we could not let her die, but we also understood that we couldn't give her the inner recourse she needed.

The greatest tragedy of all was that Susie's condition just couldn't be helped. We were permanently waiting for the phone call to come through to say something had happened. None of us could ever fully relax. We all had that ominous sense that one day she would carry out a very serious, purposeful attempt to take her own life. Waiting was a torment that stretched out for months on end until, finally, the inevitable happened.

It was a Friday and my other daughter Rosie had been out with Susie earlier in the day and had a quiet drink with her at The Moorings pub by the canal in Leamington. Susie left early and went straight home. A few hours after she left, Rosie gave her sister a quick phone call before she herself went to bed. The phone rang a few times before she finally picked up. The noises Rosie heard on the other end of the phone were to remain with her forever. A mumbling, groaning sound echoed out of the

receiver. 'Rosie, I think I have done something silly...' came Susie's dying voice. Then there was the sound of a thud as she dropped the phone.

That night Susie had gone straight home from the pub with the intention of committing suicide. She had two bottles of wine, two bottles of Babycham and a mountain of pills. She filled one glass with the tablets and mixed it with the alcohol.

When Rosie and her friend Tania arrived at Susie's apartment, they saw a scene that was very deliberately laid out. Susie had taken a blanket and two pillows, and made her own deathbed. After taking the deadly concoction of drugs and alcohol, she lay down and waited for death to overcome her.

When the girls arrived, Susie was semi-conscious. Next to her head lay four empty bottles and she held in her arm a teddy bear that Rosie had once given her. This bear had become her best friend and she wanted it with her for this final act. Rosie and Tania tried to pick her up, but Susie was in a delirious state. She struggled furiously and kicked out when they tried to touch her. In the end, the girls had to use heavy force to get her into the car and drive her to the hospital.

Thanks to Rosie's speed in reacting to the situation, Susie's stomach was pumped before the pills had a chance to enter her system. If she had been an hour later, it would have been too late. Rosie phoned me from the hospital. It was *the* phone call I knew would come one day, yet nothing can prepare you for it.

The journey to the hospital was horrific. Obviously, I did not mind going through red lights, or breaking the speed limit by a huge margin. All I could think about was how sad and tragic Susie's life had been. The helplessness I felt was in stark contrast to everything else that was going on in my life. All the businesses I had were doing well and I had all the toys a man could want. I

had many friends and had travelled the world. Yet my daughter, who was more important than all of this, enjoyed nothing in life. I suddenly understood why she had tried to kill herself, I could see her logic. There was nothing for her in the world. After 25 years of life, all she had known was sadness and loneliness. That sudden realisation sent a wave of guilt through me unlike anything I had experienced before. The thought of Susie's despair tattooed itself on my mind and I knew at that moment my own life was going to change dramatically. I would never rest easy until I had helped her.

When I got to the hospital and went to the emergency ward where she was being treated, I stopped outside the door for a minute. I felt completely inadequate. What could I do or say, even at this time of most desperate need? Usually I can find words to help pick people up in certain situations but this time my mind was blank. There was no point in lying; there was no point in giving her false promises. She knew as well as I did that there was nothing available to make any difference to her.

'The first thing I said to Mum was, "Oh, so I am still alive then?" I could see Mum was crying, but that did not change how I felt.'

Chapter 2

WHAT EXACTLY ARE LEARNING DIFFICULTIES?

NEGATIVE ATTITUDES TOWARDS LEARNING DIFFICULTIES

Amongst the ill informed, there has always been this long-running view that problems such as dyslexia and ADHD are not real conditions. Going back to the seventies and eighties, a lot of people thought they were nothing more than excuses given by middle-class parents, who wanted their children to be high achievers.

Even today, these attitudes still manifest themselves. In November 2005, an hour-long *Dispatches* documentary entitled *Dyslexia the Myth* went out on Channel 4 in the UK. This programme attacked everybody in the learning difficulties world. It attacked teachers for using the wrong teaching methods; it attacked the Dyslexia Institute for using the wrong programmes; unbelievably, it attacked the Dore Achievement Centre saying that we had 'no research'; it attacked parents for not communicating enough with their children.

As you can imagine, it just incensed everyone. Every parent and every teacher knows that children with learning difficulties

are suffering from something very, very real. The fact that some so-called experts still refuse to acknowledge that learning difficulties have any scientific basis is scary.

I am amazed how little some people have actually thought through the problem. The fact is learning difficulties like dyslexia are real conditions. If you teach a child something and they have already forgotten it the next day, are they being difficult? Do they choose to forget what they have already learned? Of course not! It is a tragic condition and it is astounding how little understanding exists about what these children and adults have to put up with. No one chooses to be forgetful, no one chooses to be disorganised, no one chooses to find reading difficult, and no one chooses to find concentration difficult. These things are beyond their control and it is very cruel to think of them as stupid, lazy or thick.

We now know that many children with issues like Susie's are actually extremely bright. It is the level of a person's creativity that gives us a clue about their underlying intelligence. Hence, there are many famous businessmen, scientists and artists who have enormous creativity and intelligence, but struggle with the basics such as reading and writing. Indeed, you might be surprised at the number of people rumoured to have ADHD or dyslexia.

Many high-profile people are reported to suffer, or have suffered. Amongst them are Richard Branson, John Lennon, Tom Cruise, Robin Williams, Whoopi Goldberg, David Bailey, Leonardo da Vinci, Thomas Alva Edison and Albert Einstein. But for every one of these high-profile folk there are a million more with similar symptoms that do not fulfil their potential. In fact, it is clear that they frequently suffer from the depressive tendencies that so often manifest themselves alongside learning issues – and, when this is the case, it affects them seriously and detracts from their quality of life despite their outward success. If we are ever going

to move forward on this issue, it is vitally important that people understand the problem. Only when this happens can we start to develop a very different society.

PROBLEMATIC DEFINITIONS

There is no doubt that learning, attention and behavioural difficulties have been around for an awful long time. The problem has been that the labelling of the issue has been dreadfully unreliable. Some children have tended to be diagnosed according to the focus and skill sets of the professional providing the diagnosis. If that professional is more tuned to the concept of ADHD, as they are in America, then the child will often receive that label. In the UK, the same children could be more likely to be labelled as having dyslexia.

We now know that the overlap between ADHD, dyslexia and other learning or behavioural difficulties like dyspraxia and Asperger's Syndrome is huge and, in fact, they are all part of one spectrum. Thus, the whole subject of labelling needs a complete rethink for two reasons: first, labelling is unreliable and, second, we have come to regard labels like 'dyslexia' and 'ADHD' as having negative connotations. In fact, these conditions usually, but not always, hide a bright person whose intellect is waiting to be released.

As is always the case, when things get a bit medical I seek help from Dr Roy Rutherford, the Medical Director for Dore Achievement Centres, to explain them. So, for most of the following section, he must take credit.

WHAT IS DYSLEXIA?

Dyslexia literally means 'difficulty with reading'. It was originally used to describe the problems seen in neurological patients who

had damage to the language areas of the thinking brain. Indeed, in the early twentieth century, many medical specialists believed that developmental dyslexia in children who developed reading difficulties without any evidence of brain damage was a functional problem within the very same area of the brain. Only recently, with the advent of brain scans, has doubt been cast on this theory.

In 1968, the World Federation of Neurologists (WFN) defined dyslexia as 'a disorder in children who, despite conventional classroom experience, fail to attain the language skills of reading, writing and spelling commensurate with their intellectual abilities'.

In the eighties, the only definition of dyslexia was an exclusionary one. If a child's difficulty with reading could not be explained by low intelligence, poor eyesight, bad hearing, inadequate educational opportunities or any other problem, then it was determined by exclusion that the child must be dyslexic. A more specific definition was needed rather than one based on exclusion.

The International Dyslexia Association (IDA) defines dyslexia as a neurologically based, often familial, disorder that interferes with the acquisition and processing of language. Varying in degrees of severity, it is manifested by difficulties in receptive and expressive language, including reading, writing, spelling, handwriting, and sometimes in arithmetic. Dyslexia is not the result of lack of motivation, sensory impairment, inadequate instructional or environmental opportunities, or other limiting conditions, but may occur together with these conditions.

The National Institute of Health (NIH) in the USA defines dyslexia as a specific learning disability that is neurological in origin. It is characterised by difficulties with accurate and/or fluent word recognition, and by poor spelling and decoding

abilities. The NIH has spent many years researching learning disabilities. They have found that:

- Dyslexia affects at least one out of every five children (20 per cent)
- Dyslexia affects approximately the same number of boys as it does girls
- Dyslexia is the leading cause of reading failure and school dropouts in the USA
- Reading failure is the most commonly shared characteristic of juvenile offenders
- Unless helped, children do not outgrow reading failure or dyslexia.

Key features of someone with dyslexia
He (or she):

- Often has average or above-average IQ, but doesn't do as well on school tests as they should
- Feels 'dumb', has poor self-esteem and lacks confidence
- Becomes easily frustrated and emotional about school, reading or testing, and often uses avoidance tactics to get out of doing these things
- Seems to 'zone out' or daydream often, gets lost easily or loses track of time (attention deficit)
- Reads or writes with additions, omissions, substitutions, repetition, reversals or transpositions of letters, numbers or words
- Often confuses left/right, over/under
- Has difficulty telling or managing time, being on time or learning sequenced information or tasks

- Mispronounces long words; transposes phrases, words and syllables while speaking
- Often has poor working memory so finds it difficult to work things out in their heads.

WHAT IS ADHD?

ADHD was first talked about at the turn of the twentieth century. In 1902, Dr George Still, a physician with an interest in children's diseases, described to the Royal College of Physicians in London those children who seemed to him to be restless, passionate and apt to get into trouble. Dr Still suggested they had 'an abnormal defect of moral control'. He wrote an article in *The Lancet* on the subject. For a while, the condition was linked to the influenza encephalitis pandemic of 1917–18, when it was called Post-Encephalitic Behaviour Disorder.

Over the years the hyperkinetic (increased energy levels) activities were thought to be the predominant feature and the term 'Hyperkinetic Impulse Disorder' was coined in the fifties and 'Hyperactive Child Syndrome' in the sixties. *The Diagnostic and Statistical Manual* (DSM) of mental disorders was established by the American Psychiatric Association and is now a standard method recognised internationally to assess various behavioural and mental conditions. Now well established, it described the condition for the first time in 1980 calling it the 'Hyperkinetic Reaction of Childhood' disorder. Later, the emphasis fell very much in the direction of attention deficits and the term ADD was first used, defining the disorder as with or without hyperactivity and focusing on inattention and impulsivity. Further revisions defined the term ADHD, its symptoms and cut-off scores for diagnosis.

The current fourth edition of DSM criteria further split the

disorder into ADHD (predominantly inattentive), ADHD (predominantly hyperactive) and ADHD combined type (both inattention and hyperactivity). Unfortunately, too little is really understood about the brain-based causes of the condition and experts continue to argue over the underlying disorder.

There are a number of different diagnostic procedures available, none of which is 100 per cent reliable and all, until now, are dependent on subjective opinions. But modern technology is now lending a hand in clarifying the biological basis of this complex disorder. The advent of MRI (Magnetic Resonance Imaging) and functional MRI (which analyses blood flow during brain activity and can identify areas of activity during rest and when performing tasks) has lead to the observation of both structural and functional differences in the brains of ADHD subjects compared to normal subjects. The most consistent findings appear to be a reduced size of the lower mid-line cerebellum (at the back of the brain) and the mid-brain area.

In the past, it has been presumed that the problems lay with the front part of the brain. However, we believe that this is not always the case and that, in fact, in the majority of cases a person is likely to suffer because it is their cerebellum that is not functioning appropriately. Supporting this are several pieces of evidence. We know from a number of studies over the past 20 years that the cerebellum appears to be poorly developed when ADHD is present. We also know from functional scans that the cerebellum is poorly activated in ADHD, whereas in other studies there is inconsistency in the frontal lobe activity ranging from underactivity to normal activity and overactivity.

Recent research at Harvard University in the United States has shown that the drug Ritalin (commonly prescribed for its treatment) appears to increase the activity in this same area of

the cerebellum that is found to be poorly developed in ADHD. We also know that ADHD rarely stands alone as a disorder and normally exists side by side with disorders such as dyslexia, developmental co-ordination disorder (dyspraxia) and even autism. This either implies multiple areas of brain disorder or a common area of poor brain functioning impacting on all other separate brain areas involved. Some current independent research into these supposedly separate disorders now suggests a single underlying cerebellar cause. This could easily explain how these different disorders are seen together so often.

THE COMMON SYMPTOMS OF ADHD

Generally, ADHD can be divided into attention symptoms, hyperactivity symptoms and impulsivity symptoms. The hyperactivity symptoms are usually grouped with the impulsivity symptoms when being assessed.

The DSM IV criteria define nine separate symptoms for both attention and hyperactive/impulsive conditions, and that six or more must be seen to confirm a diagnosis. Also, these symptoms must occur within more than one environmental setting – for example, both at school and at home. Other requirements for diagnosis are that symptoms should have been present from before the age of seven and that there should be no other psychiatric conditions present that could account for these behaviours.

Most specialists use a 'yes' or 'no' response to each question but recently a more rigorous method has been developed which asks that the responses be graded into four choices ranging from 'all the time' to 'never'. This leads to a more sensitive measure of the behaviour problems. As yet, there are unfortunately no biological tests which can be applied to detect this disorder but this might change in the near future.

The following are the attention-based criteria used during diagnosis:

- Often fails to give close attention to details or makes careless mistakes in schoolwork, work or other activities
- Often has difficulty sustaining attention in tasks or play activities
- Often does not seem to listen when spoken to directly
- Often does not follow through on instructions and fails to finish schoolwork, chores or duties in the workplace (not due to oppositional behaviour or failure to understand instructions)
- Often has difficulty organising tasks and activities
- Often avoids, dislikes or is reluctant to engage in tasks that require sustained mental effort (such as schoolwork or homework)
- Often loses things necessary for tasks or activities (e.g. toys, school assignments, pencils, books or tools)
- Is often easily distracted by extraneous stimuli
- Is often forgetful in daily activities

The following are the hyperactivity-based criteria used:

- Often fidgets with hands or feet, or squirms in seat
- Often leaves seat in classroom or in other situations in which remaining seated is expected
- Often runs about or climbs excessively in situations in which it is inappropriate (in adolescents or adults, may be limited to subjective feelings of restlessness)
- Often has difficulty playing or engaging in leisure activities quietly

- Often 'on the go' or often acts as if 'driven by a motor'
- Often talks excessively

The following are the impulsivity-based criteria used:

- Often blurts out answers before questions have been completed
- Often has difficulty awaiting turn
- Often interrupts or intrudes on others (e.g. butts into conversations or games)

WHAT IS DYSPRAXIA (OR DEVELOPMENTAL CO-ORDINATION DISORDER)?

Dyspraxia literally translates as difficulty (dys-) with movement (-praxia). This can be evident with the large movements of arms and legs, making people appear awkward or clumsy. Sometimes, it is the small (fine motor) movements where difficulties may be experienced – for instance, pen-handling skills including writing and drawing, also sometimes called dysgraphia.

There are varying degrees of clumsiness and some children may have problems with only fine motor skill, some with balance and others with the larger movements of the limbs (e.g. awkward catching, throwing or running). Some have all these problems together. The World Health Organisation (WHO) states that it affects 6–8 per cent of all children to varying degrees, while other estimates vary between 10 and 20 per cent where diagnosis has been broader.

With dyspraxia, there is often a difficulty in co-ordinating the left and right sides of the body and between the upper and lower body. This can lead to those who have dyspraxia often avoiding sporting activities, especially if ball-handling skills are required. Sometimes, they also experience a heightened sensitivity to

noise and touch. Some children with dyspraxia can have speech difficulties, such as stuttering or slurring words when young. This is referred to as 'oral dyspraxia' or 'verbal apraxia'. Many speech symptoms are referred for speech-therapy training.

Dyspraxia is often seen in children born prematurely and results from an immaturity of brain and cerebellar development. Recent research at Kings College London and Harvard Medical School in the USA show specific developmental problems in the brain and cerebellum in premature infants. Children with dyspraxia are often said not to crawl in the usual fashion as babies. However, many seem to have quite normal early milestones such as walking.

KEY FEATURES OF DYSPRAXIA

Children with dyspraxia may exhibit the following characteristics:

- In younger children small objects can be difficult to pick up
- Unable to properly complete jigsaws/games that involve sorting
- Difficulty in holding a pencil and poor handwriting
- Cannot sort shapes or toys effectively
- Throwing and catching games are difficult
- Low muscle tone (can lead to lax joints)
- Difficulty in dressing or tying shoelaces
- Using a knife and fork is unco-ordinated
- There is confusion in laterality (telling left from right) – child changes between right and left hand, and may not develop a fully dominant side until much later than average
- Inability to recognise or predict dangers

- They can physically tire easily
- They may demonstrate general irritability or limited social skills
- There is often poor posture or body awareness
- Often poor spatial awareness
- They may give inappropriate verbal responses or seem immature
- Limited ability to concentrate
- Late development in language
- Difficulty in understanding prepositions, e.g. in/on/behind/underneath
- Unable to follow sequential instructions.

These are the most common symptoms described in dyspraxics. Some are rarer than others are; some of course are also elements of other problems like dyslexia or ADHD.

WHAT IS ASPERGER'S SYNDROME?

The term 'Asperger's Syndrome' was coined by Lorna Wing in a 1981 medical paper. She named it after Hans Asperger, an Austrian psychiatrist and paediatrician, who published a paper in 1944. His work was not internationally recognised until 1990 – yet another example of how important breakthroughs can often be ignored.

Asperger's Syndrome is a milder variant of autism. Both Asperger's Syndrome and autism are, in fact, subgroups of a larger diagnostic category. This larger category is called either Autistic Spectrum Disorders (ASD) mostly in European countries, or Pervasive Developmental Disorders (PDD) in the United States (DSM IV). In Asperger's Syndrome, affected individuals are characterised by social isolation and eccentric behaviour in childhood. Individuals with Asperger's are considered to have a

higher intellectual capacity compared to those with autism while also suffering from a difficulty with social interaction. There are impairments in two-sided social interaction and non-verbal communication. Though grammatical, their speech is peculiar due to abnormalities of inflection and a repetitive pattern. Clumsiness is prominent both in their articulation and in gross motor behaviour (the way we move the limbs of our bodies). They usually have one or more areas of obsessive interest and often less than usual interest in things more appropriate and common to their age group.

According to the DSM IV guidelines, which provide the diagnostic criteria for almost, if not all, psychological conditions, Asperger's Syndrome is diagnosed by the presence of some, or all of the following behavioural characteristics:

- Lack of ability to use non-verbal communication behaviour such as making eye contact, using facial expressions and body postures in social interaction
- Failure to develop peer relationships appropriately
- A lack of spontaneous ability to share enjoyment, interests or achievements with other people (e.g. by a lack of showing or pointing out objects that may be of interest)

Also, there are typical repetitive patterns of behaviour that include at least one of the following:

- A preoccupation with one or more particular subjects to an abnormal level
- Inflexible adherence to unusual routines or rituals
- Repetitive mannerisms (e.g. hand- or finger-flapping, twisting or complex whole-body movements)

- Persistent preoccupation with parts of objects
- The disturbance causes significant impairment in social, occupational or other important areas of functioning but no significant general delay in the use of language (e.g. single words used by age two years, communicative phrases used by age three years, etc.)
- There should be no significant delay in cognitive development or in the development of age-appropriate self-help skills, adaptive behaviour (other than in social interaction) and curiosity about the environment in childhood.

As you can see, just working out which labels to use is not easy. However, it is important to remember that these are only labels and the combination of symptoms found in real life number far more than the number of labels. The fact is that labelling of dyslexia, ADHD, dyspraxia and Asperger's Syndrome has been far too rigid. The symptoms of these learning difficulties often occur together, making them extremely difficult to categorise. For instance:

- 75 per cent of dyslexics also have symptoms of ADHD, dyspraxia or both
- 84 per cent of ADHD sufferers also have symptoms of dyslexia, dyspraxia or both
- 64 per cent of dyspraxics have symptoms of ADHD, dyslexia or both

The following table looks at how conventional assessment puts symptoms into categories. However, look how much crossover there is between them:

WHAT EXACTLY ARE LEARNING DIFFICULTIES?

KEY   1 = Mild/sometimes present   2 = Common symptom   3 = Usually a severe symptom

LEARNING BEHAVIOUR SYMPTOM SUMMARY				
SYMPTOMS	DYSLEXIA	DYSPRAXIA	ADHD	ASPERGER'S
Poor reading (difficult, tiring, jump words)	3	2	2	1
Poor handwriting (scrawling, or neat but very slow)	2	3	2	2
Poor concentration	1	2	3	2
Low self-esteem	2	2	2	2
Hyperactivity	1	1	3	1
Clumsiness (catching balls, riding a bike etc)	1	3	2	3
Speech problems		1		1
Poor (short) memory (lists, names, phone numbers etc)	1	1	1	2
Poor social skills	1	1	2	2
Repetitive/ compulsive			1	2
Poor time perception	1	2	1	2
Poor emotional control (frustration, anger, depression)	2	2	2	3
Poor sleep patterns (especially when young)	1	1	1	1

29

LEARNING BEHAVIOUR SYMPTOM SUMMARY

As the table shows, there is so much overlap between the conditions that the practice of dividing them into separate categories is slightly misleading. The fact is people with learning difficulties often share very similar symptoms. All too often in the past people have simply been labelled according to which symptoms are more noticeable. If you had problems with reading, then you were dyslexic. Trouble sitting still? You were hyperactive. Couldn't catch a ball? You were dyspraxic! However, it is not nearly that straightforward.

Our theory is that all learning difficulties are the result of the same neurological problem in the brain – caused by a delay in the development of the cerebellum. These problems are interrelated and affect some people more severely than others. They are all caused by the inability to learn, or automatise certain types of knowledge or skill. This particular neurological condition will be looked at in more detail in the next chapter. However, for now it is worth pointing out that this is an issue far more common than has ever been imagined. Many, many people suffer from this problem and most do not even realise it.

For instance, look through the list below. Do some of these symptoms sound familiar? Of course, no one suffers from all of these problems, but many of those who suffer from several of them are needlessly underachieving. Before looking at the list, remember that Cerebellar Developmental Delay (CDD) is not a disease. It is not of itself painful, nor is it life threatening. It is simply a delay in the required development of one area of the brain. If we were all tested for CDD, an amazingly high proportion of us would be found to be affected to some degree. Each of us knows that there is nearly always one area where we personally find the development of certain skills more difficult

than average – for example, we may have some, but not all of the following features during development:

- Slow to learn to ride a bike (*see also* clumsiness)
- Difficulty in learning to tie shoelaces
- Difficulty in learning to tell the time
- Poor sleep patterns
- Problems differentiating between left and right
- Problems with sequencing, e.g. sorting coloured beads
- Problems differentiating between 'in' and 'out', or 'up' and 'down'
- Tendency to jumble phrases and words
- Stammering
- Difficulty in learning rhymes
- Difficulty clapping in simple rhythm
- Late speech development
- Walking quite early, but not necessarily crawling first
- Difficulties getting dressed
- Preferring 'junk' foods or covering all food with ketchup

In social situations, we may have some, but not all of the following:

- Poor organisational skills including forgetting things, living in a mess
- Difficulty establishing friendships
- Insensitivity to other people's feelings
- Difficulty in showing affection
- Difficulty maintaining eye contact
- Tendency towards impulsive behaviour

- Inability to be satisfied, and always looking for more stimulation
- Tendency to talk incessantly and repeat things
- Difficulty in following directions
- Poor spatial awareness
- Inability to process thoughts and feelings quickly
- Difficulty in expressing yourself
- Poor short-term memory – remembering phone numbers, names, lists, etc.

In school and college work, there will be some, but not all of the following:

- Problems with, and lack of interest in reading – often jumping words
- Poor spelling and putting letters and figures the wrong way round
- Difficulty remembering tables, alphabet, formulae, etc.
- Poor handwriting, including leaving out letters or putting them in the wrong order
- Difficulty in writing on the lines
- Problems with writing and getting work completed quickly
- Mixing upper and lower case in words
- Inability to sit still or concentrate on one task
- Difficulty in concentrating
- Problems processing language at speed
- Confusion with places, times and dates
- Difficulty with planning and writing essays
- Difficulty processing complex language or long series of instructions at speed

- High achievement in one or two subjects, but very poor in others
- Increased likelihood of experiencing bullying
- Tendency towards truancy

Then, in emotional life, some, but not all of the following:

- Significant tiredness after school or work
- Tantrums when faced with complicated instructions, or difficulty doing simple tasks
- Low self-esteem which, as you get older, can sometimes include suicidal thoughts
- Fear that you are as lazy or thick as you are told you are by others
- Sense of isolation
- Frustration and anger often caused by an inability to put things in context
- Irrational phobias
- Tendency to be moody

In sport and physical activities, some, but not all of the following:

- Little interest in sport, especially team sports, but some have great skills in skiing, surfing and rollerblading
- Very good at some sports and very bad at others
- Clumsiness – inability to catch, or to kick balls
- Bumping into things
- Poor posture
- Odd gait or clumsy, uneven way of walking or running

In working life, some, but not all of the following:

- Poor sequential memory – inability to sort and remember information
- Poor handwriting
- Poor concentration
- Difficulty in writing long reports
- Inability to prioritise tasks
- Tendency to be indecisive

Researchers at the Dore Achievement Centres believe that if a person suffers from several of the above symptoms they may be suffering from CDD. For us this is a far more appropriate way of defining learning difficulties than using the labels 'dyslexia', 'ADHD', 'dyspraxia' or 'Asperger's Syndrome'. CDD focuses on the root cause of learning difficulties and is not inappropriately associated with being thick or lazy. Other definitions tend to focus on symptoms such as poor reading and writing to define whether a person is dyslexic or dyspraxic. Yet, as we have seen, these symptoms refuse to sit neatly in rigid compartments. In other words, a person with ADHD may have similar symptoms to a person suffering from dyslexia. A person suffering from dyslexia may have co-ordination problems in the same way as a dyspraxic person, and so on.

The overlaps between the traditionally defined conditions are never-ending. Therefore, it may be time for all of us to start thinking about learning difficulties in a completely different way. Instead of trying to understand them from an outside perspective (i.e. if that person cannot read, he must be dyslexic), we should consider them in terms of a neurological condition. We should think about learning difficulties in terms of the root cause and we should focus on the significant potential awaiting discovery.

Chapter 3

MY STORY

I imagine my life is similar to many of those who grew up in the Welsh valleys in the forties and fifties. My family were very much working-class and my father did a variety of selling jobs and drove around in a little Austin A30 van, which was his mobile office. My mother was a secretary in a local factory and gave birth to me in a cottage a couple of hundred yards from a great castle called Castell Coch. I was born at the southern end of the Taff valley, north of Cardiff, in a beautiful village called Tongwynlais. I lived in a small cottage without electricity. The toilet was 30 yards down the garden and the *Western Mail* was behind the pipe for toilet paper. It was a simple life without the modern luxuries that today we take for granted. If I wanted a bath, I would have to go three miles to my grandmother's house in Nantgarw.

From where we lived, the vista was magnificent. You could see across to Radar and the Dolomite mines. You could also see the huge viaduct that spanned the valley, under which a wartime pilot had once flown a spitfire in a bid to show off to his friends. We

eventually moved to another house in Tongwynlais, but the view from our new home was no less beautiful. The top end of the garden looked out towards the coast and I would sometimes sit out there for hours trying to catch a glimpse of the sea.

I was extremely happy and proud to be Welsh. As a child, I was able to walk through the woods and along the disused railway line without any fear of danger. My friends and I would often stuff ourselves on the wild strawberries and berries that grew in plentiful supply in the summer. It was a beautiful and tranquil place, and it was a safe and exciting environment in which to grow up.

Yet, despite my fondness for my country, I only ever managed to retain a few words of my native tongue. I learned these in a school play and I remember them until this day: '*Beth sydd bod hen wraig? Pam ydych chwi crio?*' Roughly translated, this means 'What's the matter, old woman? Why are you crying?' Of course, in those days Welsh was not taught anything like as much as it is today.

In 1959, my parents moved us to Coventry because there was more work there. I was nine at the time and I remember initially hating city life. In Wales, I had been able to go to the top of my garden to get a magnificent view towards the sea. I was fortunate to gain a scholarship to King Henry VIII School on the outskirts of Coventry at the age of 11 and was lucky enough to receive a fantastic education. However, as I went through school, my ambitions for what I wanted to do became more and more vague. I had a notion that I might like to be a management consultant, but hadn't the faintest idea what that entailed, or how to become one. Although I did reasonably well in my O-levels, by the time I reached my A-levels I had lost all interest in studying and I knew there was no way I was going to get into university.

The only thing I was sure of was that I had an interest for business. When I was 14, I started my first venture in photography with my cousin, Colin Davis. We took pictures of families, weddings and children. Goodness knows why anybody would want to commission a youth to take professional photographs! It was lucky for me that they did as it paid my pocket money handsomely during my school years, so much so that by the age of 17 I was the proud owner of a blue Ford convertible, albeit a slightly rusty one. I was also developing a great fascination for computers, which in those early days of the 1960s they needed to house in huge air-conditioned rooms. This interest eventually led to my first proper job. After a very disappointing set of A-level results, I went to work for Jaguar Cars in Coventry, where I stayed for five years. It was an exciting time to be involved in computing and, as was the case for everyone in this new profession, I got an enormous amount of responsibility thrown at me for my age.

But it was at the age of 23, when I decided to leave Jaguar, that you might say my entrepreneurial spirit truly kicked in. I think I probably am entrepreneurial, although I am still not sure what the word really means. Some people think it is mainly linked with risk-taking. However, I have always taken it to also mean being hungry and driven to develop some product or service that is better than everyone else's. As both apply to me, I probably would describe myself as an entrepreneur. When I see something that is desperately needed, that everyone is saying cannot be achieved, I get excited. It can take over my life and drive me; it gets me out of bed in the morning with a spring in my step.

When I left Jaguar, I saw an opportunity and a need in fire protection, and suddenly I could think about nothing else. Every waking hour I devoted myself to it; I even dreamed about it. In 1974, there was new legislation having an impact (the 1971 Fire

Precautions Act), which made it compulsory for guesthouses and hotels to make many changes to their buildings to satisfy fire safety requirements. I could not see any organisation that was geared up to meet this need and so it seemed very natural to me at the time to start my own business.

There were only two slight problems with my reasoning. First, I was only 24 and I did not have a clue about how to start a business and, second, I knew nothing about fire protection. Nevertheless, I decided it was an opportunity I could not miss and within months I had negotiated some huge contracts for my company. Looking back now, I must admit it seems so strange. I myself would not do business with a wet-behind-the-ears 24-year-old. To put it mildly, I had extremely good fortune and it was not long before I spotted an even more promising opportunity for the fire protection of structural steelwork. At the time, mineral fibre and cement-based products were used and were aesthetically dreadful. I knew that if you could find some hard, decorative way of providing fire protection to steelwork then it would be a major improvement. After researching the issue, I discovered a fire-protective paint that was to transform my business and my life.

Although I did not realise it at the time, I had actually taken on a pioneering role in trying to solve a massive problem that the world had; indeed, a problem that is still evident today. We all watched with horror when the World Trade Center collapsed in 2001. This happened because the steelwork in the building had become so hot that it lost its strength, leading to the collapse of the structure.

These days, many of the world's biggest structures use the fire-protection technology that my company, Nullifire, was championing 30 years ago. At the time, of course, the Establishment was absolutely against the paradigm shift we were

driving, saying things like, 'it won't work', 'it cannot happen', 'there is no legislation to support it'. Goodness knows why, but none of this fazed me. I never really thought about failure, it did not even come on to my radar screen. I guess when you are walking the tightrope everything is fine, providing you do not look down. Indeed, I never looked down, I was not even conscious that there *was* a down. As far as I was concerned, this was something the world needed, so I was going to give it to them. In the end, the product was a fantastic success and it resulted in architects having the opportunity to design large buildings in a much more attractive way. Most of the recently built sports stadia and airports now use this technology.

One thing I learned from those early days was that it is an awful lot easier to sell a concept if someone has done the legwork before. When you are the first person to come up with an idea, you have to try to educate people about the concept and possibilities. This is a long, slow and hard, but ultimately worthwhile, process. Every day all around us we see this sort of thing happening. A hundred or more years ago, if you had gone to an optician with the concept of laser eye surgery, you would have been laughed out of the building. Today, it is becoming standard practice. In the same way, the structural fire-protection methods I pioneered in the mid-seventies have become standard practice around the world today.

Without a doubt, the work I did in my early career geared me up for what I am doing now; it was a great foundation for me. I have been down this path before and I know that the concepts about learning difficulties our team of experts have been developing will one day become the established view just as the discoveries we made about fire protection did. Indeed, as you will discover in this book, this process is already taking shape.

INVOLVEMENT IN EDUCATION

In 1999, a friend of mine came to me and asked if I could help get his child's school out of financial difficulties. That school was Arnold Lodge School in Leamington Spa, which had an excellent reputation because the class sizes were small and the teachers so caring and competent. To me, it seemed tragic that my friend's son, who had been born with difficulties and had needed a series of operations, would have to leave a school that he loved. Thus, I started negotiations to buy it.

As soon as my cousin, Gareth Newman, heard about the plight of the school, he also expressed an interest in helping and so we bought it together. This sort of altruistic gesture was typical of a man who had dedicated his whole life to helping others. Out of all the people I have met in education, Gareth is one who has greatly inspired me. He is a dedicated man who sees potential in children and would obsessively focus on helping them until he had exposed that potential. At one time, he was the youngest headmaster in Britain and subsequently had a number of headships before finally being asked to develop Corby City Technology College on a green-field site. This Institute achieved phenomenal success in helping children, and Gareth's efforts were rewarded in 2000 when he was given a CBE for his Services to Education.

I think watching Gareth at work gave me hope that there might be more skill and ability in everyone, especially those labelled 'thick' or 'stupid'. At the time we were developing Arnold Lodge School, I asked him how he had made such a difference for the children in Corby. He told me one of the most important things he discovered was the importance of encouraging children to set their own targets. Instead of being told what they needed to achieve, they felt a sense of ownership about their

own progress. The other thing he said was important was the regular measurement of their progress so that both children and teachers could see what they were achieving, which they find remarkably motivating.

One day, I put it to him that, if we developed a simple online system to do exactly what he described and that all teachers could use, surely his methods could be made available nationally and help large numbers of children achieve their potential.

Following this conversation, we put together a plan to develop software that could be used to help assess children on a national scale. The dream was that we would create online tests that would be multiple-choice and fun for children to do, whether or not they were learning impaired. This would give teachers extremely important information about how they were doing compared to national averages. It was great fun working on these projects and we managed to make the assessments really enjoyable for children to do. The software developers built in some great features, including each child being able to sit a unique test. The teacher could then use this tool as often as needed to identify all the areas where each child was weak, so that they would know exactly what to teach. It also made a graph of the progress to show the real contribution the teacher was making, which was very rewarding to the often undervalued work of the teacher assigned to lower-ability groups.

As a bonus, we found children with weaker reading and writing skills showed their true ability, as multiple-choice questions more accurately identified their actual level of knowledge in the subject being tested.

Another feature we built in, probably triggered by my concern for children with learning issues, was that, if a child was struggling to answer the questions, the computer would simplify

them so that the child did not become stressed or discouraged. Conversely, the particularly bright child, without realising it was happening, might well have the level of the assessment taken up a notch if all the answers in the early stages were being answered correctly. Thus, within minutes of the completion of this instant-access system the teacher would have a full audit of the knowledge and needs of each member of the class. What a way to drive progress in the classroom, and what an easy way to bring out the best in each and every one of a large class! Not only did Gareth and I get a real buzz out of it but so did the children we worked with using the product we finally called GOAL – Global Online Assessment of Learning.

So the first challenge we had was that the Labour government at that time had made wonderful promises about how rapidly they were going to connect all schools to the internet with broadband connectivity. We soon realised that, as is often the case, they did not always live up to their word and it would be several years before every school had the capability to use the products we had developed. But what also surprised us was how scared some teachers were to try a new concept. Many resisted it as they had their tried and trusted methods for assessing children, which, in our view, gave them very little valuable data to help them steer children through the learning process.

Nevertheless, the company continued to grow and went on to become Educational Development International (EDI plc) and merge with the London Chamber of Commerce Examination and Industry Examination Board (LCCIB). It has since become part of Pearson plc.

In 2005, the school that had made the most progress in the country – the Holy Family Catholic Primary School in Addlestone, Surrey – was using the innovative assessment product for

schools, developed by EDI. It gives me great satisfaction to know that teachers and students love using this tool to set targets and evaluate their progress. I really hope it catches on everywhere.

EARLY ENCOUNTERS WITH LEARNING DIFFICULTIES

Although when I was growing up I do not recall the words 'dyslexia' or 'ADHD' ever being used, I can now remember clearly that there were many children in my school who did have the symptoms. These children were sometimes lonely and had low self-esteem. Even though many of them were bright and creative, they simply could not get to grips with basic tasks like reading or paying attention. Of course, the notion that these people might have had a neurological problem never crossed anyone's mind in those days. Consequently, many children I knew spent the early part of their lives being bullied and ridiculed, not just by their fellow classmates but by adults as well. There was a complete lack of sympathy and it was quite naturally assumed that they were thick or lazy.

Looking back, I still feel an extreme sense of guilt. I remember one lad in my class who could not grasp the difference between years and months. When he was nine years of age, the big joke in the school was to ask him how old he was, to which he would always reply, 'I am nine.' Then, if you asked, 'Months or years?' he would usually reply, 'Months.' He was a constant source of entertainment for everyone. We would laugh ourselves senseless and hardly considered just how miserable we were making him.

I also remember a number of boys in the school who would make any excuse possible to avoid doing the physical education classes. This was not because they hated sport, but because, at the age of 11, they still could not do their shoelaces up properly. A ten-year-old boy called Mark was so embarrassed about this that

he used to come to gym class with his shoes already tied up. He would try to slip them on without anybody noticing, but, unfortunately for him and much to the amusement of everyone else, they would constantly slip off because they were not tight enough. The teachers did not have a clue that this boy simply could not learn how to tie his shoelaces so he was punished and, on one occasion, made to write out lines. Unfortunately, Mark also had a problem with his handwriting so, in the end, for him school was one long succession of punishments. I cannot imagine what he must have gone through, it must have been horrendous.

Until my daughter Susie was diagnosed with dyslexia in 1980, I had never heard about it. Once the concept was explained to me, however, it made sense and it was a great relief to hear that she was not simply stupid. Of course, no parent ever believes this of their child, but it was still a great feeling to have an expert tell me there was a name for her problem. Surely, I thought, if the enemy can be seen, it could be defeated, too.

Chapter 4

THE SEARCH FOR A SOLUTION

As Susie was slipping further and further into despair, I was reaching a new phase in my own life. My business career had been great fun and I had now reached the stage where I could afford to slow down just a bit. I had people running things for me in my various businesses and I was looking forward to spending some time on my yacht in Spain.

Yet being idle is something I have never been very good at. I desperately need to feel that creative buzz you get when you are working on something new and uncharted. Without that, everything just seems to drag along and I become extremely restless and it's hard to muster the energy to get up in the morning.

Of course, with Susie in such a bad way it was impossible to relax fully. She was always somewhere in my mind and, even when I did manage to switch off and relax occasionally, I would inevitably end up thinking about her. After her third suicide attempt in 1997, I knew I had to drop everything and devote

myself to helping her: I had the time, I had the resources, and I had the mental energy to do something. Yet, whenever I sat down and tried to think about what to do, I had no idea what else to try. Already I had spent the last ten years trying to help her. Nothing had worked and there was nowhere to go. My other daughter Rosie used to say that it would just be a matter of time before we would receive a dreaded phone call about another attempt.

Although I did not want to admit it, I agreed with her. Susie had already told me she did not want to live in this world. When someone is so miserably focused on ending their life, there is not much you can do to stop them. If tragically she had succeeded in her quest for self-destruction, I would have been devastated, but not surprised.

As often happens in these cases, when I least expected it, the answer I had been searching for finally came. In 1997, I had been in Hong Kong on business and I was standing around in the airport waiting for my plane. Roaming around the terminal, without any particular objective, I found my way into a bookshop. I remembered that I needed to replace a copy of a book a friend had given me. The book was John Gray's *Men are from Mars, Women are from Venus* and, with such a long journey stretching out in front of me, I thought it would be worth a read on the flight. Eventually, I found it on the shelf. Right next to it was another book called *Smart but Feeling Dumb* by Dr Harold Levinson (1988), and I know it sounds cheesy, but I was really struck by the title. Somehow, I sensed that I would not be walking out of the shop with just the John Gray classic.

By this point, I had already read many books about learning difficulties. I would normally get a few chapters into these books before realising that the authors were not going to offer any help

for the kind of problems Susie was suffering from. Nevertheless, reading the inside cover, there was something about the book that compelled me to purchase it. Sitting on the plane, I did my normal routine of taking sleeping pills, which ensure I get several hours' sleep and I sank back into my seat.

I love long-haul journeys as they allow me to completely switch off and get the sort of sound sleep I never seem to enjoy at home. If you asked me to choose between my own bed and an airplane seat, I'd go for the latter option every time. On this particular occasion, I thought to myself I'd just spend a bit of time glancing through this book, then I'd get some kip... As I started to get into the book, I became less and less interested in getting any sleep at all. I found myself sitting upright in the seat and feeling more and more alert as I turned every page. What I was reading spoke to me in a way unlike anything I had ever read before. It was almost as if the author knew my daughter Susie personally and was describing the exact symptoms she was suffering from. The way he described the problems, frustrations and personalities of people was like reading a summary of Susie's life. For want of a better word, it was spooky.

I have no idea what happened to those sleeping tablets because they had no effect whatsoever. As we made our approach into London, I completed the final chapter. When I put the book down, resting it on my knee, it was as if someone had turned the light on in a very dark room. All I could think about was that I wanted to contact Dr Levinson and get Susie across to see him. I believed this was finally someone who had a clue about Susie's problems and might be able to help her.

Once I had landed, I immediately started to make phone calls trying to find out all I could about this guy. Most of the people I spoke to had absolutely no idea who he was. The few who had

heard of him were not encouraging and advised me to look elsewhere. Yet all I could think was that here was a man who had been treating learning difficulties for 30 years and his ideas resonated with me. Every time I closed my eyes I thought about the things I'd read in his book

Trying to make up my mind about what to do next was a perplexing process. The next few days were spent doing intense research into Levinson's practices. I contacted many of his patients who said some very positive things. On the other hand, I also spoke to some researchers who were less enthusiastic. In fact, they were positively discouraging his findings.

After mulling it over for a while, I decided I would have to investigate the subject far more deeply if I was to draw my own conclusions. After a few more days of sitting at my computer, I noticed how most of the criticism focused on the fact that there was no scientific research to support what he was doing. I have to be honest and say that this was not an issue that greatly concerned me at the time. The truth is I was a desperate dad and I wanted a solution for my daughter – I was prepared to take a risk if it might help her.

MEETING DR HAROLD LEVINSON

I knew there would be a problem persuading Susie to come with me to New York. In the past, I had taken her to meet so many doctors and specialists and each time her hopes were dashed. As I did not want this to happen again, I decided to take a different tack. I told Susie I wanted to take her on a shopping spree and that it would just be her and me. I expected this would strongly appeal to her because she would not have to fight for my attention. When we were on the plane, I casually brought up the fact that we were also going to pop in to see a specialist who

might be able to help with her reading. I did not make a big deal out of it and, as far as she was concerned, the whole trip was about us spending some quality time together.

Of course, inside I was bursting with anticipation. When we finally got to Dr Levinson's building, I remember feeling ever so slightly disappointed. I had expected some type of huge Manhattan-style building. After all, if this clinic truly was offering Americans a breakthrough treatment, surely it would be located in impressive surroundings. Instead, what we entered was a perfectly professional, if somewhat small, building that was neither in Manhattan, nor in the slightest bit grand. First and foremost, it was a place of work and I felt that it had 'small scale' written all over it.

The staff, however, made up for any disappointment I might have initially felt. They were kind and helpful, and added a great deal of clarity to Susie's situation. I felt a huge amount of relief that someone at last understood the issues Susie was facing. They dealt with every single one of my many questions that I tirelessly and endlessly fired at them. I wanted to know if Susie's condition would be permanent, I wanted to know if they had met anyone else like her, and I wanted to know if they thought their treatment could help her.

The whole time the one thing that kept burning in my mind was the fact that reading issues are a global problem affecting at least 10 per cent of the world's population. If this was truly *the* groundbreaking cure everyone was looking for, then why had the government not made it available across the country? For that matter, why did they only have one tiny clinic in New York?

Later, I found the answer in another book written by Dr Levinson. In *Dyslexia: A Scientific Watergate* (1994), he describes

the enormous problems he had in trying to get his work accepted. He also talks about the hatred and professional jealousy that filters through the whole industry and an absence of an altruism that would be helpful to finding a solution. In such a competitive atmosphere, the chances of any researchers or experts working together to develop a cure are reduced. As my background had been in the building-products industry, which was typically dog eat dog, you would expect me to be pretty well versed when it came to this sort of conflict. However, reading his book, I could see that in the field of learning difficulties the tensions and rivalries were even more intense than those I had been used to.

When we finally met with Levinson himself, the first thing he wanted to do was carry out a range of tests on Susie. At the time, I thought they were very strange indeed. These included a balance test to see what her co-ordination was like. He also put her on a spinning chair and then tested her eyes.

In the space of two or three hours, he did a number of other neurological tests to help build up a complete story of her. He then prescribed for her a very complicated cocktail of drugs and nutrients. Susie was told she would have to take these tablets every few hours for the coming months. She was also given a chart showing her the increasing drug doses she would take over a period of time.

Susie, of course, was completely numb to the whole experience of being tested. She just wanted to get the whole process over as quickly as possible and go shopping. Following the consultation, she was neither impressed nor optimistic. However, she agreed to start the programme as soon as we got back to England.

ON LEVINSON'S PROGRAMME

Within weeks of the start of the treatment, we began to notice a difference in Susie: it was obvious something was happening. Instead of running straight up to her room as soon as dinner was over, Susie seemed to be taking more interest in conversing with her family. It was thrilling to see her able to do things with which she had struggled before. As her abilities grew, so did her self-confidence, and for the first time it seemed that she was finally on track to some sort of recovery.

It was steady and slow progress, but it *was* progress. In fact, the change that took place in Susie was more dramatic than anything any of us had seen before and it was not long before we all became converts. What amazed me most was that it was plain to see that, even though Levinson's theories clearly had some merit to them, no one seemed to be listening to him. For 30 long years, he had worked as a lone researcher. To me, it seemed scandalous that because of an academic conflict a whole generation of people had failed to benefit from this new treatment. So began the challenge of my life. I wanted to help develop further and spread what Dr Levinson was doing. Little did I know what I was letting myself in for...

THE RESEARCH PROJECT

From the discussions I had had with various academics, it was clear that if this treatment were to gain credibility it would need huge amounts of research to back it up. Not being a researcher, I had no idea how to do this. Nevertheless, it did not take me long to find out what needed to be done. I then phoned Dr Levinson and asked if he would allow an independently monitored research project in the UK. I told him that, with the permission of the parents, the research project could be carried out in Arnold Lodge

School. It was not by any means a 'learning difficulties' school, but like every school in the world it had its fair share of children with such difficulties. Within a few months, Dr Levinson flew his family, his staff and his equipment to the UK.

The first thing that I arranged was for him to give a talk to parents at the school. He spoke about his theories and ideas, and told them stories about case studies. The talk was so successful that within a few days not only did we have all of the equipment set up, but we also had about 50 parents wanting to sign their children up. These students were put on the course and it was agreed that they would be assessed over a period of six months.

It is interesting to note that at first there was a lot of concern amongst the staff, who were worried that Arnold Lodge would be seen as a 'special needs' school. The school itself had built up a very prestigious reputation and so in some ways it was not surprising that there was a lot of nervousness surrounding the project. Nonetheless, the stigma attached to learning difficulties has always frustrated me and even back then I knew it was something that must go. Even so, I gave all the staff assurances that the school would not turn into a learning difficulties school – rather the opposite, in fact.

The research project went ahead and over the next few months we saw many interesting results. The teachers noticed that children on the course were becoming less disruptive in class as well as being more retentive. Parents were also happy because they saw that their children were starting to enjoy school more. The longer the tests went on, the more signs there were that what we had in our hands was a potential treatment that could turn around everything people thought they knew about learning difficulties. Everything was looking very positive and, as time went on, I began to feel more at ease.

THE ONE DRAWBACK

During all this time, Susie continued to make progress. However, the drug regime was quite long, complex and difficult to follow, and I was getting a little concerned that the dosage of amphetamines was increasing frequently. I began to ask more and more questions about when and if Susie would be able to come off the drugs. Worryingly, all of my questions were answered very vaguely and so I decided to ask other patients how long it had been before they had finished the course. The answers I received were also vague and inconsistent, which started to worry me even more.

Any responsible parent reading this might think I was foolish to keep my daughter on the programme. However, for all my doubts the one undeniable fact was that Susie had made some progress. Years of trying different methods had not had anywhere near the impact on her life that Dr Levinson's drugs programme was having. It was for this reason that I had faith in what we were doing.

STAGE TWO: GOING IT ALONE

Within a few weeks of the completion of the research project, Dr Bonnie McMillan, the independent educational psychologist researching the treatment, came to me with the results. They were significant and remarkable. Finally, we had the independent research we needed to help us start to challenge conventional wisdom. I was also over the moon: Susie and 50 others had now made some headway in overcoming one of the most blighting and misunderstood conditions of our time.

My first reaction was to phone Dr Levinson and offer him substantial financial backing to open around ten clinics in the UK using his methods and name. My plan was that we would open these clinics in a short space of time and carry out another larger

research project. In my view, if we could do this successfully, his methods would be developed and refined further so that ultimately what seemed to be an effective solution could become universally accepted quickly, and we could start making a real difference to thousands of people's lives.

Overnight, Dr Levinson thought about my proposal and called me the next day. To my great surprise, he told me that he did not want to work with me because my background was commercial and not medical. I found this a bit strange as I was offering to contribute a lot of money and I was not asking for any return on it; I simply wanted to make his ideas universally acceptable very quickly. Nevertheless, as I imagine many highly respected scientists do, he had a deep suspicion of the commercial world. Seeing my whole background had been in business and was not in the slightest bit medically based, he decided he would be better off without me. He probably assumed that I wanted to exploit his work and make as much money as possible. In fact, I had no need for money and my motives were, and still are, genuine. I simply had a very strong and personal interest in seeing this thing through to the end.

The criticism of my commercial background had no impact whatsoever on me. I knew that my care and concern was about Susie and all the other Susies in the world. Within seconds of his refusal, I had already decided that I would go it alone without his help. Looking back, this parting of ways was certainly the key turning point in the eventual development of our research. Had I gone on working with Dr Levinson, I would probably have been constrained to include working with prescription drugs. Now, starting from a clean sheet of paper, I sensed there might be a way of producing something even more effective with no potential side-effects.

The complicated combination of drugs and nutrients that had been so key to Dr Levinson's treatment had always troubled me somewhat. Just like many psychiatric treatments used to control a condition, once you stop taking the medicine, the benefits stop, too. While I was delighted with its impact on Susie's behaviour, I was also aware that it might not be a long-term solution. I knew Susie could not rely upon it forever, and I did worry that there might be some side-effects. In this sense, it was not the cure I had been looking for.

Even so, I will always be grateful for the light Dr Levinson shed on Susie's problem. Without his research, I may never have understood why she found it so hard to learn and the breakthrough subsequently made may never have happened.

Chapter 5

THE BREAKTHROUGH – AND HOPE

It is funny how sometimes in life you meet people who say very little and are relatively understated but, when they do say something, it is priceless. These people have the ability to impart sheer wisdom and can flip your whole world with a simple utterance. Professor Rod Nicolson of Sheffield University is one of these people. In one simple turn of phrase, he gave me the answer I had been looking for. His inspired genius was to lay the foundation pillars for our whole treatment, and who knows? Had he not given me the inspiration, the programme we have now may never have been developed.

Professor Nicolson had spent many years researching the cerebellum. One of the main problems he faced was that the theories developed by Dr Levinson had not been well received by his fellow practitioners and any time the cerebellum was mentioned it was met with a knee-jerk reaction. Nevertheless, Professor Nicolson had done some impressive scientific work illustrating the connection between the cerebellum, automatised skills and cognition.

The path to finding a way forward was by no means clear. In my mind, I had a very definite picture of what I wanted to achieve. My ideal was to develop a permanent, non-drugs-based solution for Susie's reading difficulties. However, I had no idea how I was actually going to do this. It was only in 1998, after Professor Nicolson uttered an inspired pearl of wisdom, that a plan began to form. During one of our many discussions, he mentioned that 'anything repetitive might lead to a change in the cerebellum'.

On the journey home from our meeting, I puzzled over what he had meant by this. If you could change or develop the cerebellum with 'anything repetitive', surely there might be a new way of tackling learning and other behavioural difficulties just waiting to be discovered? Eventually, I called him and we discussed the issue further. I asked him if lots of different repetitive exercises could have an effect on learning. He said that, in theory, they could, and that was that. This germ of an idea became the basis behind much of our research strategy.

PUTTING THE JIGSAW TOGETHER

Around the time of Dr Levinson's project in England, I desperately needed a UK doctor who could supervise the prescription of drugs, and make sure everything complied correctly with the guidelines of the British Medical Association (BMA). I had spoken to many doctors but had not found anyone willing to take this on.

Thankfully, there was one man who, after a bit of arm twisting, listened to what I had to say. Dr Roy Rutherford was a thoughtful and well-respected doctor, who I was lucky enough to know socially. He was the sort of doctor who, despite my lack of a medical background, would debate medical issues with me, which made him an invaluable friend. Grounded and solid, he was not held back by any preconceived ideas. I made no secret of the

fact that I really needed his particular skill set on board for this adventurous project – this was no ordinary venture. Yet even the open-minded Dr Rutherford must have found my early assertions somewhat preposterous. What I was basically saying was that virtually the whole medical and educational establishment had been on the wrong track as far as the treatment of dyslexia and ADHD were concerned.

I obtained some basic information on Dr Levinson's methods and gave them to Dr Rutherford for him to evaluate. As you might expect, being a consummate professional, his enthusiasm was initially quite a bit lower than my own. In fact, reading over the documents I had given him was hardly high on his list of priorities, which for a while frustrated me. However, when he heard about my proposed research project, he could see that I was deadly serious. His interest quickly grew and he became the medical supervisor for the Arnold Lodge project.

When he saw the results of the project and realised its potential in the same way as I had, he quickly became very enthusiastic. So much so, in fact, that when I parted ways with Dr Levinson and the time came to find an alternative exercise-based cure, he was totally committed to being involved. His role was to look diligently and thoroughly into every aspect of research around the world and to pull together the many hundreds of pieces of the scientific jigsaw.

Pioneering work by Jeremy Schmahmann of Harvard Medical School, research by Rod Nicolson and Angela Fawcett of Sheffield University, and lots more was unearthed and pieced together into a large jigsaw of knowledge. With each new piece Dr Rutherford dug up, he gained a clearer picture of how to tackle this massive issue. He seemed to have this innate ability to read huge complex research papers and make clear, sensible logic out of them.

What's more, he seemed to enjoy doing it. Often, he could hardly hide his excitement. Even to this day, he will often run into my office and breathlessly expound yet another piece of research that he has uncovered that adds even more support to everything we have been doing.

As Dr Rutherford went through more and more of these papers, he found that many of the pieces of the jigsaw puzzle we needed were already there. We were not the first people to discover that exercises can stimulate the brain. Not only did he need to assimilate all this knowledge but also to fill in all the gaps, too. After all, we were looking for a permanent solution for learning difficulties. We needed something that would make a complete and long-lasting difference to people's lives.

During this whole process, Angela Fawcett gave us more clues. Working with Rod Nicolson, she had been evaluating the way in which the cerebellum is responsible for what they termed 'automaticity'. This refers to the way the cerebellum develops skills into an automatic processes. As an example, think about how you write with one particular hand – a very complex process – without thinking about every move you make. By contrast, when you write with your other hand, it is slow, scruffy and far from automatic.

Another major breakthrough came when we started to look closely at the pioneering work done by physiotherapists in the rehabilitation of cerebellar stroke victims. This work involves the use of specific exercises that had the effect of helping to reduce the symptoms suffered by patients in the aftermath of a stroke. Some of these exercises were to provide the ideas for developing our earliest research programmes.

So it was largely thanks to Professor Nicolson's ideas and Dr Rutherford's assiduous research that we started to piece together what might be a road map to lead us to a solution. The

complete answer to finding a cure for learning difficulties was still a long way off, but I was beginning to feel quietly optimistic about the future.

Thanks to these breakthroughs, we managed to dream about a non-drugs-based treatment, but now we had to find a way to make this a reality. The one thing that was becoming very clear was that in order to treat a person with learning difficulties we were going to need highly specialised equipment. This would help us to pinpoint the area of the brain that was underperforming because it was underdeveloped.

We turned to all the relevant manufacturers and many of them gave us demonstrations, but nothing we were shown was suitable, or accurate enough, for our purpose. Weeks went by, and more and more salesmen came pitching their products to us. I felt completely frustrated until the very last sales representative pointed me in the direction of someone he said might be able to help me.

Rachel Smith was a researcher working on a project in the Channel Islands. She specialised in audiology and she seemed to be exactly the person we needed. When I phoned to offer her a job working for me, she thought I was joking. I assured her that I was genuine and told her all about our plight, and how we had not been able to find the right equipment. Within two weeks, she was part of our team and we sent her off to America to try to succeed where we had so far failed.

Rachel drew my attention to the fact that reports of some space missions mentioned many astronauts suffered symptoms that, to us, appeared to be a temporary form of dyslexia. Maybe it was as a result of this that NASA had been involved in the development of a machine to help identify the cause of these problems.

I sent a six-figure sum to have this equipment bought and

shipped over from America for us. The destination on the delivery address was a garage in the courtyard of my house, which was exactly where we were to set up our first clinic.

One of the key things obsessing us at the time was how we were going to interpret the results from the equipment and turn them into specific exercise programmes. Throughout this time, many other things really puzzled us. We could not understand why so many seemingly bright people struggled to concentrate – and often with relatively simple tasks like reading or expressing their thoughts in writing. Nor could we understand why so many people displayed such a wide variety of symptoms – there are a large number of symptoms and they turned up in endlessly different combinations. Therefore, we took to testing everyone that we could possibly persuade to come and try this new-fangled equipment – we needed research data and we needed some guinea pigs! Looking back, we laugh a lot about those we persuaded to try it. We tested everyone from the local butcher, the local publican, the housekeeper and her husband to professors and teachers. I think we only just managed to stop short of putting Sally, the family dog, on the equipment.

Like many people, I have never really understood how my own mind works, so trying to understand everybody else's was a huge task. However, after testing many hundreds of people we were starting to see some pattern in the results. Susie was just a typical, though extreme, example of the many we tested with poor reading skills. What amazed me more than anything early on was that we discovered that virtually no children or adults with reading difficulties had been able to learn the skill of moving their eyes smoothly from one side to the other. This ability is, of course, fundamental to reading and it shocked me that this fact was not generally known.

The next step was to develop a set of exercises capable of overcoming these eye-tracking problems. At this stage, we thought that one day we might be able to provide a simple generic set of exercises that could be printed in textbooks used all over the world. However, it gradually became evident that this would not be possible because everyone displayed their own set of symptoms, a consequence of how the infinitely complex wiring in our brains has formed, giving each of us the unique aspects of our personality and character. We therefore started to experiment with a series of exercises that could be individually tailored to people's needs, guided by the results of the neurological tests we were doing to establish where in the cerebellum there seemed need for further development.

THE FIRST CASE STUDIES

What an exciting time that was! A myriad of research projects were going on simultaneously and I hardly had time to stop and think about what we were achieving. Already, we had established the area of the brain that seemed to be responsible for causing all of these symptoms. We had also managed to obtain and adapt the equipment for identifying the neurological problems and were beginning to develop exercises capable of starting the remediation process.

It dawned on me that I had one almighty challenge ahead of me that I had not considered. How on earth was I going to be able to convince people to spend 10 to 20 minutes a day trying out some exercises for up to a year when, at that time, there was no evidence, let alone a guarantee of success? Even for Susie, who was now an adult, there was no certainty that in her chaotic life she would ever be able to do the exercises in a consistent way without significant supervision. It was obvious that I would

initially have to find people willing to make one huge leap of faith to take on the programme at all.

By this point, I had already become a bore at every wine bar that I visited, and for whoever I sat next to when I travelled on a train or on a plane. I was constantly talking about learning difficulties and the things we'd discovered. Nevertheless, not everyone found what I had to say boring. I soon discovered that I was very far indeed from being the only parent with a child who had suffered greatly.

The more I talked about it, the more I realised that everyone I met knew someone who suffered from a learning difficulty. There were myriads of sick-with-worry parents who had no idea where to turn. I looked to this group for my early research subjects and presented to them, such as I could, our research and theories.

I was fortunate enough to find a few volunteers who were desperate for any help available and willing to try anything. The cost, of course, was the commitment that they would need to do exercises twice a day, every day for a year. The fact is that this was no simple task. Even in the most organised of families, just finding an extra five minutes in the morning and in the evening is not always an easy task. Nevertheless, they all gave me a firm commitment that they would follow the programme to the letter.

So, with what now seems like a primitive set of exercises we started our research. Initially we tested the exercise programme of three subjects. Susie was the first person to go on the programme in April 1998 and Simon Wheeler (not his real name) and Jamie Frances followed her shortly after.

SIMON WHEELER

When he started the programme, Simon was 13 years old. The only son of parents living in a nearby village, his mother had long

been convinced that Simon was very bright and very able, and yet this certainly did not show in his schoolwork. She had tried to persuade the Local Education Authority to give him the support he needed and, as is so often the case, she had an enormous battle on her hands. However, her determination paid off and they helped put Simon into a boarding school catering for the needs of children like him.

Despite the best efforts of his teachers, Simon made slow progress. He seemed to have little ability to retain information. Once it was inside him he could process it, but getting it in there in the first place was a real problem. Simon suffered from the same personality traits as many who have learning difficulties. His self-esteem was not very high. In his early teens, he was not confident enough to take the local bus into town to see his friends. His concentration was poor and he found it draining to focus on homework. In sport, he had some potential in golf and, aided by his father, he had been given a handicap by the age of 13, which he was particularly pleased with. However, he did not find other sports so easy and for him life really wasn't a very pleasant experience.

Even though our programme was at a very early stage of development, Simon's mother was eager to get him started. It was obvious that she was exactly the kind of mum who would ensure her child did the exercises twice a day, so I was happy to include him.

JAMIE FRANCES

Jamie was the son of the family who owned the local garage and filling station. He was at a local school with a very good attitude to learning difficulties and he was taken out of maths and English lessons to be given one-to-one attention. Despite this, he still had

many problems and was not improving academically. He also had problems with his co-ordination, making him poor at sports. For him, this was a particular embarrassment because he had two older brothers who were both very accomplished sportsmen.

His parents were not prepared to consider putting their child on a course of drugs and were at a loss as to what to do next. When I heard about Jamie, I offered to put him on the course. Although he was a shy child, like Simon, he had a delightful attitude and a good nature, and I really wanted to help him.

We tested these early research cases every few days, adjusting the exercises and looking for changes. Little did we realise what a massive task it would be to work out which exercises could influence which area of the cerebellum and then to deduce which exercises might make the condition worse rather than better. Nevertheless, as great as the challenge was, the encouragement we were getting was equally compelling. As we continued to experiment with different types of exercises, it became more and more evident which ones were having an effect.

The most obvious way in which we were able to measure this was through the changing attitudes of the parents. As their sons went through the programme, Simon's and Jamie's parents went through a series of distinct shifts in attitude. When they first came to us, they were understandably and realistically cynical about the programme. It couldn't have helped matters that the whole operation had been set up in my garage! Once the testing had been done, however, and we were able to show them the reasons why Simon and Jamie had learning difficulties, they began to show signs of confidence in what we were doing, although this optimism was naturally peppered with a healthy dose of scepticism. A few weeks later, when Simon and Jamie were starting to show some signs of improvement, their parents went

through a third stage; one of sheer optimism and belief. They began to realise that all the changes they were seeing were not coincidences: the programme was working.

The changes we saw in the two boys were quite remarkable, but you can read more about this in a later chapter. In the meantime, you may be interested to read a speech Jamie Frances has just made at the time of writing, five years after he was one of those early guinea pigs!

At a conference in Leamington Spa on 14 March 2006, Jamie gave this speech:

I am truly delighted to be here speaking to you this evening. I have come to speak about my life-changing experience that would not have existed without Wynford. Through his help and pioneering work with the Dore equipment, I was able to develop a range of skills which I had never dreamed of and fulfil some of my greatest dreams and ambitions.

From the age of about five, I was diagnosed with serious dyslexia. I found being dyslexic very hard. It was pretty much impossible to concentrate so my learning was very slow. I had to battle through, just scraping along at the bottom of the class. I did, however, receive a lot of help from teachers but they dealt largely with the symptoms rather than the cause and the strategies they put in place were of limited value. It did not seem fair that I would try so hard and get nowhere – it was like coming home really hungry and having to eat your dinner with chopsticks for the first time, every time. This caused me much distress and anger; all I wanted was to be able to do things that everyone else could do so easily. I wanted to

be able to catch a ball or play sports without my teammates being disappointed that I was in the same team as them. This regularly drove me to tears and the only thing that kept me going was the support that I got from my loving family, who kept me motivated and guided me in the right direction.

My life took a huge turn when I received a telephone call from Wynford, asking me whether I would go round to his house on Friday evening to be assessed on some new equipment that he'd got. I found the equipment rather odd at first but by my second visit I was starting to get used to it. On the third visit, the equipment had been moved to an outbuilding of Wynford's house, of which my main recollection was the bitter cold. I was set some exercises to do with beanbags, which I really enjoyed. We did them as a family and had huge fun with them. Each week I really enjoyed being assessed as I felt I was able to do things better and better. I soon became able to play tennis, which I loved, and I even began beating my brother, which was fantastic. My memories of the clinic were very positive and I would get told that I was getting cheekier each time I went. My ability to concentrate grew more and more, and my confidence in myself increased massively. After a short time at the centre, my learning-support teacher invited my mum and dad to discuss what had happened to me. Never in her career had she seen someone improve so much in such a short period of time. I had gone from a reading age of a ten-year-old to that of a 15-year-old, and I was still only 14½.

I cannot stand here and list everything that has improved in my life – if I did, you would need to bring a sleeping bag! My sporting success was amazing as I began

running competitively for Warwickshire Schools. I then started a sport for which I have developed a great passion – rowing – and within two years I was ranked third in the country in my age group. This seemed so extraordinary because just a few months ago I found any sport extremely difficult, especially one that involved co-ordination. Yet now I was living for sport and loving school, too.

I will never forget a comment that a teacher once said to me in Year 6 at primary school. She said, 'You would be lucky to make your GCSEs.' Six years later, I was stood on stage at Kineton High School as head boy giving a speech on student life. As I stood addressing the audience, I noticed a face in the audience which I recognised. I carried on and just finished. I noticed she had a tear in her eye and it became strikingly obvious that this lady was the teacher who told me I would be lucky to make a GCSE. I was immensely proud as I stood there partway through my A-levels having been voted head boy of the school.

I have now finished my A-levels and have been offered places at a number of universities, where I plan to go and study Sports Coaching and Sports Psychology. I am currently the youngest qualified junior rowing coach in the West Midlands. In addition, this Easter I have been invited to coach at a National Junior rowing camp designed to nurture other young gifted and talented athletes.

The Dore Centre has made me a much more ambitious person and has equipped me with the necessary skills to go on to follow my passions and fulfil my dreams. Most of all it has boosted my self-confidence beyond recognition, giving me the personal drive to aim for my goals and not let anyone put me down.

Every single one of you in this room is extraordinary. Without you, other dyslexic people like me will not have the door unlocked to all those beautiful opportunities that are open to me. You hold the key to that door and have the power to add so much value to so many people's lives. I remain forever grateful for what Wynford has done for me and can only urge everyone here to continue helping him unlock other people's dreams.

While Simon and Jamie were flourishing, you might be wondering what had happened to Susie...

SUSIE AND THE PROGRAMME

It was clear that Susie had not enjoyed some of the experiences of the programme of drugs she had been put on. She had been taking ever-increasing dosages and there seemed to be no end in sight. On several occasions, she had tried to wean herself off them, but sadly this resulted in withdrawal symptoms, which alarmed me greatly. I was therefore very keen for her to try this new treatment and had my fingers crossed that it would help her.

But things did not start off smoothly. Within 24 hours of Susie being put through the tests and given the exercise programme, I realised there was no way she was going to voluntarily stick to it. Everything she has previously tried to do had failed, so why bother with this? I then started a pattern of ringing her several times a day and badgering her until she began to do them more consistently. However, once she got into the swing of it, we started to see some subtle changes.

The most obvious change was that she was so much happier. At the time, we were just beginning to understand the relationship between her many troubling symptoms and auditory

and verbal skills. It was becoming clear to me that a major cause of low self-esteem could be the direct impact of slow verbal and auditory processing. Susie's inability to think quickly enough meant she had real problems conversing with those around her, especially in group situations. Consequently, she spent the majority of her life feeling negative and down about the world.

Watching her struggle her way through social situations, while having to constantly put up with the sneers and slights, had been extremely painful for me. What a wonder it was then to see her finally emerging from within herself and participating in social interactions. She was even beginning to initiate them herself. When I observed her having a conversation, I could see the comprehension in her eyes. She did not look tired and stressed any more, and there was an air of calm about her: she was easily processing all the things being said to her, understanding them and responding. It felt like watching someone who had mastered the art of playing a musical instrument. No longer was she hitting the wrong keys, or playing out of time. The conversation was flowing briskly and naturally. More importantly, I could see she was starting to enjoy every moment of it.

The progress Susie was making was also in basic skills. I must stress that her case was considerably worse than most of the people who now go through the programme and realise great benefit. Her problems were extremely severe, meaning that, even though the most basic reading skills had been hammered into her after much private tuition and schooling, she was still many years behind where someone of her age should have been. Although we never specifically gave her any further teaching while on the programme, there was a very sudden, unmistakable improvement. It was almost as if all of the teaching she had received over the years was finally beginning to process in her

mind and the fog around her eyes starting to lift. Although she did not become a bookworm overnight, she was beginning to pick things up and read them, which was thrilling to watch.

One of the most enlightening moments came not long after she had started the remediation programme. Uncle David, or 'Uncle Dai' as he is known by our family in Wales, was a very popular member of the family and he had died in 1999 after a long illness. On the way to the funeral, Susie sat in the front of the car, which was a marvel in itself because normally she would be at the back with her headphones on in her own lonely world. On this occasion, she started talking about what a wonderful man Uncle Dai was, and what she had learned from him. It was very out of character to hear her talking like this anyway, but, when we were half an hour into the journey, she said something that made my eyes pop out of my head.

Susie began discussing the thoughts and feelings that must have been going through Uncle Dai's head when he was enduring so much suffering at the end of a long and happy life. She started to talk about whether or not euthanasia would have been appropriate for his condition. When she said the word 'euthanasia', I glanced up at my rear-view mirror and saw her brother and sister looking back at me with their mouths wide open. They both pointed at Susie and made a gesture as if to ask 'what on earth has just happened?'

The fact that she knew the word amazed me, that she could say it staggered me but it was frankly unbelievable that she put it in the correct context in a sentence. For the first time in her life, Susie was talking with great clarity and intelligence. For all of us, it really was an earth-shattering moment. It was as if suddenly her impairment had gone and, with it, her loneliness had disappeared.

We have now worked out that Susie always had the intelligence and the thought to match, but did not have the processing capacity to share it. No wonder she was so frustrated.

OPENING OUR FIRST CENTRE

As you can imagine, word was beginning to spread. Every parent wants their child to be happy and bright because they know this will unlock a treasure trove of opportunities for them. They always hope that one day their real potential will shine through and they will go on to achieve great things. It is extremely difficult for any parents to watch their child struggle with learning basic or essential skills and continually fall behind academically, often to finally retreat into themselves socially. For many of these parents, this remarkable new programme was a last resort – a final gamble to try to give their child the chance of a normal life. Within a few months, we had more and more people knocking at our door wanting to participate in the programme. With my cold, drafty garage no longer a viable option, we moved the clinic into offices in Leamington Spa. The building was actually an old school, so we aptly named the centre the 'Old School Clinic'.

The opening day at the centre in 2000 was a very exciting one. For me, it was a venture into a new era and there was a real buzz amongst the dedicated team of researchers who had worked so hard to make this day possible. Even though emotions were flying high, the day went extremely smoothly. When the press arrived, they seemed much more impressed by the fact that some of the equipment had been originally developed and used by NASA than they were by the life-changing results we were getting. They were also impressed, of course, by the anecdotes of many of the parents and patients who had taken a gamble on the programme. Now they were talking excitedly about how it had changed their lives.

I will never forget the scene of the numbers of proud parents standing by their children who, just a few short months ago, had all sorts of challenging symptoms. Now these children were making rapid progress at school, catching up with their peers and, for the first time, enjoying their school life. Their mums, dads and teachers had always realised they had more potential and finally they had been proved right. For many it was a dream come true. One of those parents, who happened to be a head teacher, brought tears to my eyes when she told me that *I had given her back the child that she had always wanted*.

So it was not long before we outgrew our office in Leamington and had to move into even bigger offices in Kenilworth.

When I started researching the programme, my initial reaction was that I should do it through a charity. This was because the driving force behind the programme was to put something back. However, because our ideas were relatively new and we did not have the backing of the Establishment, I was told we should not try to go down this route. We were doing things few if any of the researchers in this area would support. Given that charities generally are only allowed to do things that are supported and not permitted to do anything financially risky, we would have to consider other options. Therefore, I did the only thing I knew how and developed the programme through a commercial company, which is allowed to take such financial risks.

Little did I imagine the countless times I would have to explain my motives in doing this. So many people have criticised our efforts because they see our programme as a moneymaking scheme. This is wrong on two counts. First, to date, it has cost me virtually the whole of the fortune I have made to develop the programme. Second, my only motive was to save my daughter's life – not to make money.

One of my next challenges was to plan to make the programme accessible and affordable to the millions who needed it, something that remains an issue until governments, through education or medical departments, provide it free of charge. Here, there were many issues with which to contend. The first problem was that the equipment needed was very specialised and extremely expensive; the second was that it required highly trained specialists to operate it.

This second problem was not so easy to solve. There were not enough appropriately skilled specialists in the world to meet the demands of so many with learning and attention issues. There was no way I would be able to find and train hundreds of them. As you can imagine, we were also on a very steep point of the learning curve and constantly coming across new ideas and data causing us to rethink and fine-tune many of our assumptions and thus change the programme. Up to this point, our resident audiologist had been Rachel Smith, who had skilfully kept our system updated and relayed any updates to our close-knit team of professionals. Now it seemed inevitable that we would be taking on hundreds more, who would see thousands of people go through the programme. Trying to keep them up to date with the latest test criteria and exercises while maintaining a high level of quality was going to be a logistical nightmare. There is no establishment turning out professionals with the combination of skills required by our programme.

We were soon joined by Carolyn Dando, an excellent researcher whose skills have contributed to the development in so many remarkable ways. The good fortune we have had in finding such competent and highly motivated staff still amazes me to this day.

So, as is often a case when there is a lack of sufficient

expertise, I did what any like-minded professional would do and looked to developing very sophisticated software to clone the expertise of people like Carolyn. This would have the effect of simplifying the whole process so that we would not actually need those rare skill sets to operate the equipment, as the software would make all the important calculations necessary for prescribing an exercise programme for an individual. The skill sets of our therapists would, therefore, need to be based around communication and motivation rather than technical and medical techniques, which would be dealt with by the computer program.

The only way forward, therefore, was to develop and make our own purpose-made equipment. During the coming months and after the development of several generations, we finally settled on a very sophisticated and intelligent version and put it through the exhaustive process of CE marking and FDA approval. This whole process was costly, but well worthwhile in that we ended up with equipment that was reliable, safe and producing very accurate results. We had created lightweight, low-cost equipment that could be cost-effectively transported and used around the world. Now nurses, physiotherapists and teachers who go through a short training programme can use the equipment. One advantage we did have in 2001 was that internet technology was becoming widely available. This meant that the process of linking testing equipment across the world up to a single computer server would be comparatively easy.

Thus started the most absurd development project I have ever been involved in. I had given myself the challenge of developing software and equipment more sophisticated than anything I had ever seen before in any medical establishment; I had engineers and software developers led by Peter Yates, a young software genius, working unrelentingly against the clock to get everything

ready. Somehow, despite the furious nature of this development, they managed to rise to the challenge. The software they developed was not only a valuable timesaving tool, but also instrumental to the whole future of this project. We ended up with a system that could be used anywhere in the world by a whole range of professionals who wished to be trained up. At the same time it meant that we had created a global data collection facility other organisations could only dream of.

I must admit that it winds me up a bit when people say the organisation is a commercial venture. The fact that the company has made huge losses seems to have been missed by some people. The reason we charge at all for the programme is very simple. Without government backing, we needed some sort of contribution to enable us to help thousands and at the same time collect sufficient research data to influence the authorities. If I was Bill Gates, then maybe I could have afforded to help a few million more; as it is, I was only able to subsidise a few thousand to complete the programme. Had I been taking a salary, had we been making profit, I guess my conscience would not be so completely clear. As this is not the case, it has enabled me to robustly answer that small number of critics who, interestingly, all seem to have a vested interest to defend. I truly am sorry they feel threatened but my greater allegiance is to those we want to help.

Before closing this chapter I should mention that at the time of writing the situation has now changed somewhat; we have been instrumental in setting up a charity called The Dore Foundation to research how cerebellum-based theories can reach everyone who needs help. There will be more on this later in the book.

Chapter 6

THE THEORY BEHIND
THE PROGRAMME

First, let's remind ourselves that what we are sharing with you is a theory. However, recent scientific discoveries have enabled us to use this theory to provide a clear explanation for so many symptoms of learning and attention problems. We now firmly believe that they are all caused by a delay in the development of part of that area of the brain called the cerebellum (CDD – Cerebellar Developmental Delay, a term coined by us during our research). Thus, in order to know how our programme works, you must first learn a bit more about the latest understanding of how the human brain works.

THE CEREBELLUM
There are two main areas of the brain that we are concerned with – the thinking brain (or the cerebrum), which deals with thought processes and language, and the cerebellum, located at the base of the brain.

Until recently, the cerebellum had not been studied anything

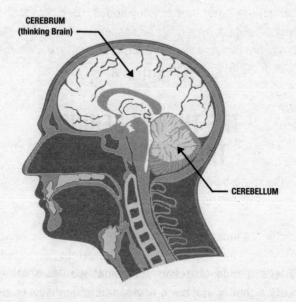

CEREBRUM
(thinking Brain)

CEREBELLUM

like as much as the thinking brain, but now we know it has a very important role in influencing the way we function. Though it is only the size of a small orange, it has as many neurons and cells as all the rest of the brain put together.

It is the cerebellum that co-ordinates so much of what we do every day including:

- Co-ordinating and helping us to retain information as we receive it
- Controlling our limbs
- Controlling the fine movements of the eyes, hands, mouth, tongue and vocal cords
- Co-ordinating our balance
- Linking the 'feeling' or 'emotional' parts of the brain to everything else that is happening

If the cerebellum is not properly developed, then the control and co-ordination of fear, anger, happiness, etc. may be impaired.

When we are carrying out a task of, say, writing, the cerebellum is the part of the brain that:

- Enables us to form and remember how to spell the words
  Controls fine movements with the pen
- Finely controls our eye movements for tracking words on a line
- Enables us to balance to sit up
- Allows us to concentrate and to stay on task.

You can see it is indeed a very important part of the human brain. Recent research has established that the cerebellum's ability to co-ordinate all these functions depends upon how well each individual part of it has been developed. If any part is of it is underdeveloped, the functions that that particular part controls will always be working less effectively and automatically than they should be. When people display such symptoms when writing, for instance, it causes an 'overload' in the brain's processing capacity and reduces the cerebellum's ability to co-ordinate other functions that may appear perfectly normal in other circumstances.

It is remarkable how many children sent by a parent to collect a list of things from upstairs have difficulty remembering the items and return with at best just one or two. Many children with learning or attention problems have a poor short-term memory anyway, but the extra demand of, say, an underdeveloped balancing process while climbing the stairs seems enough to reduce the memory capacity to the point where they can forget all the things they are trying to retain.

THE CEREBELLUM AS LIBRARIAN

One of the best ways of understanding what is happening is to think of the cerebellum as the librarian for the brain. The librarian's job is to co-ordinate all the information coming and going – the knowledge, the skills, the concepts and the memories. It must ensure that all this information is put away in the right place and that it is indexed properly so that it can be easily retrieved and cross-referenced. In other words, it must ensure the information is learned or, in other words, automatised. This applies to every type of knowledge and skill, whether it is academic, like times tables, or social, such as learning the appropriate way to react in a given social situation; it helps us recall someone's phone number and how to find our way to the supermarket.

When parts are underdeveloped, our librarian seems very capable of learning some types of subjects and hardly capable of retaining others. The subjects the librarian is interested in are properly filed away and indexed – but others are looked after in a far from satisfactory manner. Ironically, it seems likely that those with certain parts underdeveloped may well have other parts very highly developed. Could this explain why, often, those who are intellectual struggle in some way with tasks that may seem like common sense to most people?

When functioning properly, the cerebellum has to index knowledge and skills so that they can effortlessly be recalled for use and, if necessary, then be cross-referenced to other information in the brain.

INDEXING

So, the first role of the cerebellum is to index skills in the brain so that they may be called upon and retrieved automatically at any given moment. For many people with specific learning difficulties,

this basic process never fully takes place, for certain everyday skills. For example, while the rest of us can pick up a book and read it, some people with an incompletely developed cerebellum find that the simple function of moving their eyes from right to left, to enable them to read easily, never becomes automatised in their brain. Consequently, for many, reading is a difficult, slow and painstaking process that can leave them feeling tired and often very frustrated, too.

To better understand this, it is worth thinking more about the concept of 'automaticity'. When something is difficult, it often means that the skill in question has never become automatic for you. The first time you learned to drive a car, all of those knobs, levers, switches and pedals may have seemed a daunting and confusing mess. As you jumped and jerked the vehicle up and down the road, the prospect of ever being able to get your head around everything seemed impossible. However, after you have driven for a while, all those things on which you had to concentrate so hard in the early days suddenly seem to fall into place. After that, whenever you get in your car you can drive off without any trouble at all. You do not need to think about which pedal you are using, how to steer or how to use the gearstick because they have all become automatic processes.

Another example, which is very useful when trying to describe automaticity, is the process of writing. I am right-handed so when I write with my right hand I do not think about it, I just do it without any effort of concentration. I have learned that skill and it has been indexed properly and hardwired into my brain, so that when I want to use it, the words just flow across the page. However, if I try to write with my left hand, it is much harder work; I have to tell my hand where to go. A very slow, hard scruffy process can end up looking like Susie's handwriting used to when

she was younger. Again, this is because the process of writing with my left hand has never been automatised. For Susie, the process of writing with either hand did not become automatised at all until she started the programme we developed for her.

CROSS-REFERENCING

The second function of the cerebellum is to help cross-refer knowledge with other knowledge. In other words, after it has indexed away bits of knowledge, it must be able to retrieve them and compare them to other pieces of information. For the librarian to do this effectively, there needs to be lots of wires, or neural pathways, between the different areas in the brain. If these wires do not exist, our librarian's job will be almost impossible.

For example, when we meet someone at a party we may not be able to remember their name. This is because we do not have the wiring to link automatically the image of a person's face and their name. The two bits of information are stored in two separate parts of the brain, and without the wiring it is difficult to make the connection. A person may have great linkages in some areas, but poorer ones in others. For instance, some will have wonderful linkages to enable eye and foot co-ordination, but have problems in other areas like the fine motor skills necessary for neat handwriting.

The spectrum of people suffering from an absence of specific linkages in their brain varies enormously. It is rather like having big rooms in a house. Either you have connecting doors and corridors between those rooms, or you don't. If you take the case of the classic dyspraxic person, they will struggle to link what they are seeing with their eyes with the movement of their hands and their feet; those functions have never become automatically linked together.

At the far end of the spectrum, you have savants, an extreme form of autism, where individuals have phenomenal knowledge and can remember virtually every fact thrown at them. However, that knowledge just exists in seemingly isolated pockets and they are incapable of relating one piece of information to another. *Rain Man* is a film based upon a true story of a savant who had amazing abilities, such as remembering every zip code in the United States, but he also had a total lack of ability to co-ordinate simple tasks like being able to dress himself.

The theory about how we are wired does help to explain why some otherwise brilliant people make very silly mistakes. The truth is the more creative and intelligent the brain is, the more likely there will be some weakness or other. The bigger the brain, the busier the librarian is going to be.

Take the classic example of the archetypal professor who, of course, has an eccentricity. Often, we will have heard of, say, the professor who is brilliant at nuclear physics, but completely unable to learn how to change the tyre on his car. In the same way, the professor who is wonderful at philosophy may have never learned how to organise his diary. We may call them 'eccentric', but what does this mean? According to our theory, an eccentricity is a lack of ability to learn or co-ordinate certain types of knowledge or skills within the brain. The professor of nuclear physics may be unable to learn how to change the tyre on his car and the professor of philosophy may be unable to learn how to organise. These are learning difficulties, although we probably do not usually describe them as that. You either have the wiring to co-ordinate skills from different areas of the brain or you do not – precisely the developmental issues that our treatment identifies as needing attention and helps remediate.

THE BRAIN'S PROCESSING CAPACITY

It is important to note that, just because a certain skill is not yet automatic, this does not necessarily mean that you cannot do it at all. What it does mean, however, is that performing that skill will be slow, tricky and probably tiring. If I concentrate hard, I can write with my left hand, but it takes me a long time and the results are messy. In the same way, if a child has a problem such that his eyes have difficulty tracking words on a page from right to left it does not mean that he is unable to read. What it means is that some of the processes used during reading have to take place in what may be loosely called 'working memory' because those processes are not hardwired to be carried out automatically.

For a person with learning difficulties, the processing capacity or working memory is usually cluttered with tasks currently being carried out; they would not have to be performed in this sort of manual way had the cerebellum been able to automatise them. For example, if I learn a new skill like riding a bike, the chances are I will need to think very hard about balance, both during and for a while after I have learned that new skill. I would therefore be using up lots of the brain's processing capacity during this period. However, eventually the skill would become automatised and my working memory freed up so that I can ride effortlessly without thinking about it.

A person with dyslexia or ADHD will not have the luxury of lots of spare processing capacity whenever they are carrying out certain everyday tasks. Their spare capacity will be filled up quickly every time they try to listen to someone speak or try to read. Despite having had years of practice at these things, they have never become automatic.

If you are constantly filling your processing capacity with non-automatised things that really should not be there, it means you

will have a restricted ability to cope with multiple tasks. This can mean that things like remembering lists are difficult for you because you will not have enough storage space left in your mind. It also can signify, of course, that your attention span is going to be short. For example, if I have a very small amount of capacity available in my brain and I am trying to learn from a book, then I have to concentrate hard to stay on task. If someone were then to walk into the room and talk to me, the chances are that, by the time I have turned my attention back to my book, all the things I had been trying to remember would have been completely displaced. There is insufficient memory to allow me to retain the information while, at the same time, to allow me to also focus on the temporary distraction.

By contrast, if I have lots of capacity available and free, the situation would be different. If a person came into the room, I would be able to just park my thoughts in a spare area of memory and deal with the distraction. Once the person had left the room, I would easily be able to access my temporarily parked thoughts and return to my work.

POOR VERBAL VISUAL AND AUDITORY PROCESSING

So many things are taken for granted. We take reading for granted, we take listening effortlessly and comprehending easily for granted – for many of us these things are indeed effortless, but for some it is a process that has never become automatised, and just listening and concentrating becomes tiring. We call this condition attention deficit and, sadly, often those who suffer from it are called lazy, when in fact they have to work much, much harder to concentrate than those who do not have the same problem.

For some, the process of speaking is not fully automatised.

They know what they are thinking, but turning those thoughts into speech is a process that requires much more effort than it should do. Those of us who have never had this problem will really struggle to comprehend just what tragic consequences this can have on someone's life.

For others, processing what they see with their eyes is not automatic. In other words, they have to struggle to make sense of visual information and store it in the brain. We believe that all of these symptoms are caused by poor development in the cerebellum in the specific areas controlling these respective functions. Sadly, for many with common types of learning difficulties, these crucial everyday skills are not automatised.

Parents and teachers often say that, if a child with a learning or attention difficulty is focusing on one thing, such as a computer game or a television programme, they can seem deaf to the outside world when spoken to. What is actually happening is that the child's processing capacity is so full of the auditory and visual processing required by the game or TV programme that they have no capacity to also process what someone is trying to say to them, too. Their ears hear it, but they have no capacity to process it. Therefore, we should remember that, when a child has poor attention, it is often because they have to work so hard just to listen and then turn what they have heard into comprehended thoughts. This is a painful and tiring process; they are not being difficult or lazy.

This auditory processing problem is quite common amongst people with learning difficulties. For most of us, the process of hearing something and comprehending it is a hardwired skill in our brain that happens automatically when someone speaks to us. However, if the cerebellum has not indexed this skill properly, then a lot of difficult processing will have to be undertaken to turn what we are hearing into comprehended thought.

Likewise, a person with learning difficulties will sometimes also have a problem with the speed of how they process what they wish to say. This manifests itself as a delay during the conversation while they work out how to express themselves. Crucially, we sometimes say that 'we can see the cogs whirring', as the processing takes place.

THE TRAGEDY OF POOR VERBAL PROCESSING

Having to use working memory to cope with non-automatised verbal processing can cause a noticeable time delay that can be very detrimental in a person's life, particularly in social situations. Imagine a six-year-old boy with learning difficulties in a playground at school. He might be standing around with a group of children who are chatting and having a real laugh. Desperate to contribute to the conversation, the little boy will be concentrating hard on what the others are saying. However, by the time he has worked out what they are saying and then worked out what he wants to say, the conversation will have moved on a few sentences. If he decides to pipe up and say what he is thinking, he is likely to be ignored or, worse, ridiculed by other members of the group, who realise he cannot keep up with their banter.

This is a tragic and very common situation. These children often and very quickly develop low self-esteem and become isolated. They are not so bad in a one-on-one situation because the person they are speaking to usually has the patience to wait for them to express themselves. However, in a group situation, such instances of kindness rarely happen. A group of children, or indeed adults, will often not be sensitive to whether someone is processing quickly or not and, in the end, that child will feel left out of the group.

At this point, that little boy has two choices. One is that he can become a bully and use his might and muscle to demand

attention and orchestrate things. That way, he does not need to listen. The other one is to go off to the corner of the playground and pretend he is happy playing by himself. Whichever option he chooses, he will still have to endure the daily humiliation of being made to feel thick or stupid in the classroom. The scary thing is after a while he may even start to believe it.

So many kids, my daughter included, end up asking, 'Why am I different? Why do not I have as many friends as everybody else?' No one is able to explain to them why this is; all they can do is help to prop up their confidence. Some may tell them that, if they work hard to be more conscientious, their life will improve. Yet, however hard they try to do this, throughout their life they will always encounter the same problems. People will sneer and jibe that they are inarticulate and forgetful. Employers, too, will see them as inefficient and unreliable, and they may have to go from job to job. Yet all the time they are working incredibly hard just to be able to maintain a normal life.

It is a terrible scenario to be faced with when you know that something is wrong with you, but you do not know what it is. Labels like 'dyslexia' and 'ADHD' can be helpful up to a point, but they do not explain *why* you have the problem. The beauty of recent medical breakthroughs is that finally at least the 'why?' questions can be answered.

From now on, whenever a child asks, 'Why can't I read properly? Why can't I write? Why can't I make friends?' the response no longer has to be 'I don't know'. Instead, the parent or teacher can help them understand the cause of their problems. What's more, they can tell them they may not have to live with the problem any longer. This is not giving them false hope; this is pointing them towards a method that has been shown to really work in a high proportion of cases.

Chapter 7

WHY DO SYMPTOMS RESPOND DRAMATICALLY TO TREATMENT?

The treatment that has now been developed is an individualised programme that seems to tackle and improve the effectiveness of the 'librarian'. The end result is that more skills and tasks become completely automatic, freeing up the brain's capacity to process information. This is almost certainly the reason why the programme has such a dramatic effect in transforming so many people's problems.

Amongst those with learning difficulties, problems with reading are very common. About 85 per cent of sufferers show little interest in reading and, in most cases, it is because they find reading tiring and difficult. The very process of reading (if there is a cerebellum development problem) can use up lots of the brain's processing capacity:

- Controlling eye movement so that the words go in smoothly and sequentially
- Processing the meaning of each individual word

- Stringing the meanings together to enable comprehension of the sentence.

This can cause huge overload in mental capacity, with the result that reading will be very difficult, if not impossible. Imagine how this is made even worse if, on top of that, you are then asked to read out loud in class! With an already overloaded brain, this is just too much to ask and often completely impossible. For many children, this has been the cause of severe heartache and, fortunately, the practice has been largely dropped in schools today.

Poor handwriting affects 90 per cent of sufferers of typical ADHD and dyslexia, with many of the remaining 10 per cent having neat, but very slow handwriting. The process of handwriting involves very fine motor control in the muscles, an area that the cerebellum is responsible for automatising and co-ordinating. Within months of the programme starting, it is quite common to see remarkable changes in handwriting. In a recent study, one of a group of prisoners going through treatment was so amazed that his writing had improved so greatly, that he jokingly said, 'When I write a letter home now, I don't know whether to send it, or frame it!'

According to our theory, low self-esteem is a common symptom for two reasons. The first is physiological: it often takes a lot of effort for those with learning difficulties to turn what they hear into thoughts, as that audiological process has never been properly automatised. In addition, they may often take longer to convert their thoughts back into the words they want to say (verbal processing). This means that, in social situations, they find it a strain to work out what is being said and to contribute to the conversation. Sadly, all too frequently this leads to a lack of confidence. The second reason is, of course, psychological.

People affected by a poorly functioning cerebellum perform poorly at academic things, often at some sporting activities, and possibly in social situations, too, until they doubt whether they are capable of success in any area of their life!

Happily, self-esteem is often the first thing to noticeably improve when people start the cerebellar development programme. Many of those who have gone through the course experience a dramatic improvement in their social skills. This is partly because they find it easier to listen and contribute during conversations. Suddenly, they are in a position where they are no longer afraid to speak up for fear of embarrassing themselves. Not only can they participate more effortlessly in conversations, but often they initiate dialogues without any prompting: in simple terms, they start to enjoy social situations.

Poor spelling is probably caused by a combination of poor eye tracking and a reduced ability to sequence things in working memory. It affects about 90 per cent of children with learning difficulties and, of course, many adults, too. While typically spelling does finally improve after our programme starts, it is often one of the last things to show progress. If they are still being taught spellings, however, children do seem to learn much more quickly than before. Older children and adults have first to 'unlearn' their strategies for spelling before they adopt the more natural process that the programme enables.

Poor short-term memory is another problem affecting some 70 per cent of those with an incompletely developed cerebellum. Often it is seen in conjunction with impaired sequencing, or poor sequential memory, which affects about the same proportion. It makes it very difficult to remember lists, phone numbers, timetables, and so on. Short-term memory problems appear to be the result of lack of capacity in the working memory. This lack of

capacity seems to be caused by the number of tasks that fill the working memory as they have to be done manually rather than automatically. While the brain is busy carrying out these essential, but still unautomatised tasks, it is often in overload, thus reducing its ability to carry out the less critical tasks like remembering a phone number or remembering the name of the person you met last night! No wonder, then, that the consequence of increasing the automaticity of everyday functions has such an enormous impact on daily life.

Expressing 'steps' in logical thought is linked to the ability to structure sequential things. Often, people have the ability to come to an important conclusion or to make a key decision without then being able to detail the logical steps they took to get there. This is quite commonly found in very bright people who suffer with attention or other learning difficulties. For example, entrepreneurs (or other creative people) often come to clear decisions that they are quite sure about. Yet they are completely puzzled as to why these same decisions are not 'common sense' to those around them who fail to see the myriad possibilities analysed at a break-neck speed in their thinking brain.

They have used their powerful thinking brain to analyse all the options and then come to a conclusion. However, they do not have the processing capacity to work out and therefore spell out all the individual steps they actually took (probably subconsciously) in their thinking brain in a logical and sequenced way. Often, for them to structure their thoughts – whether in writing or in speech – is equally difficult. Why is it that brilliant businessmen just hate writing reports? Possibly for the same reason.

Poor organisational skills are also caused by difficulties with sequencing, and manifested in an inability to put things in the right place. Forgetting to take books to school, having a messy

desk or an untidy bedroom, slowness at getting dressed, being late for most appointments – these are all examples of poor organisational skills. To organise requires having the capacity in memory to contain several tasks at one time and reorder them according to priority or some other logical sequence. With the brain overloaded (caused by lack of automatising of many everyday tasks), it means there is simply not enough capacity to juggle things and organise them so you can imagine how much easier organisation gets when the brain is freed up.

Reduced interest in sport is partly caused by poor spatial awareness, caused in turn by poor visual processing, which leads to poor working memory capacity. For many, this means they may prefer non-team sports. For some, who in addition to their learning or attention symptoms also have difficulties with physical co-ordination, it usually means they find many types of sport difficult.

However, many with attention or learning problems find that the feelings through the feet, muscles and joints (somatosensory) are enhanced, compensating for the lack of input from the inner ear (in rather the same way that a blind person will sometimes have more acute hearing). It is for this reason that it is common to find that some are very adept at skiing, rollerblading, windsurfing, ice-skating, etc. (all sports where feelings through the joints are particularly important).

Some also prefer individual sports such as running, swimming, athletics and rowing rather than team sports. A few, however, are good at team sports but they tend to be a striker, goalkeeper or winger rather than in the middle of the team. They find it impossible to retain ball skills while having an active awareness of where other team players are and making good decisions at the same time. In these circumstances, they go into overload and

often lose their ball skills. It seems they are much more comfortable if there is one specific task to focus on – like aiming for goal! Overload in the brain's processing capacity may well be the explanation as to why so many talented players, who shine wonderfully when acting alone, lose their ball skills temporarily while under intense pressure.

It has constantly amazed us that, whether or not someone has shown any interest in sport, after the programme it is usual that many of their sporting skills will have improved, by becoming more automatic, more consistent and seemingly requiring less effort and concentration.

Difficulty with finding or following directions and a poor sense of direction are again generally due to poor spatial awareness and cause problems for many of those with ADHD and dyslexia. This is further compounded if they have difficulty reading the road signs, especially when moving, or reading maps. But it gets even worse: if they stop for directions, many have difficulty remembering sequences so that taking in a list of directions like 'Take the second left, right at the third set of lights, over the bridge, turn sharp left' is a completely impossible nightmare!

Poor concentration, often described as attention deficit is, we believe, due to overloading the brain's processing capacity. How difficult it must be to retain focus on a subject when the memory is crammed full and there is only a small space remaining for all those minute-by-minute issues that keep cropping up. In this situation, any new thing that comes up immediately displaces whatever was being concentrated on before. This problem affects large numbers of people. How cruel this condition can be! Those suffering from it are often called lazy yet they have almost certainly had to work harder than anyone else just to concentrate at all.

Tiredness after school or work is a general condition that affects about 70 per cent of those who come to us. It is possibly caused by the huge workload of concentrating, reading and writing, etc – all these functions involving mental processes that are having to be done manually (and are therefore exhausting) rather than being done automatically (and effortlessly).

Clumsiness may show itself as an inability to catch balls, difficulty with learning to ride bicycles, a tendency to bump into things and knock things over. Problems of this sort can affect between 40–70 per cent of those with learning issues to some degree or other. Some people with more severe symptoms of this type may have been labelled as having dyspraxia, or DCD. It seems that these symptoms may be due to lack of 'learning' or 'automaticity' in physical movement and co-ordination. During the programme, the typical improvement in co-ordination skills is very significant.

Showing signs of frustration and anger is a problem for about 50 per cent and it is hardly surprising if you think about it. Not only do they have to cope with the frustration of not being able to clearly express themselves or being able to do things that most other people can, but also they often have to put up with being undervalued. But there are also physiological reasons that may provide an explanation as to why such people have temper flare-ups and tantrums. Reduced processing capacity of the brain could be the reason that they do not have the space to introduce rationalising thoughts or to put the issue into context or perspective. What may well seem like small issues to most people can become big and very troubling ones for people with attention or learning issues and often they have difficulty getting over minor conflicts, taking too much to heart. Developing the cerebellum often seems to help alleviate this

distressing symptom, as it enables more processes to become automatic, thus releasing memory capacity that in turn creates space for rationalising thoughts, and so they are able to control their feelings better. Don't forget, this is just a theory at this stage, but it's one that holds good as an explanation for all the good things that we see happen when people go through and complete the programme.

Phobias may also be explained by the reduced capacity to cope with worrying things or situations. It is quite common for people with learning issues to also suffer from phobias. Being scared of the dark, of spiders, of putting their face under water... these are just some of the irrational fears patients have reported before starting on the programme. In some extreme cases, these phobias can restrict their lives, as with school phobia, or fear of open places. As the cerebellar functions improve, some find they now have sufficient capacity so they can put these fears in context and so ultimately they diminish.

Faddiness with foods – especially when young – often shows in a preference for junk foods. In other cases, there is an obsession with a particular flavour, a typical one being ketchup. We have many reports of this improving – hopefully, one day we will start to understand if this is a coincidence or not, but it seems to happen a little too often for that to be the case.

SENSITIVITY TO TOUCH

Quite a few report that young, and sometimes not so young, children with learning or attention problems feel an increased need to 'touch' items, when going through a store, for instance. Children who have this tendency are always being told off for fiddling, maybe quite unfairly, as they probably cannot prevent themselves from doing it. Others speak of unusual irritation or

sensitivity to labels inside garments. This is another area of research begging to be done. As we now believe, the cerebellum co-ordinates 'touch' sensitivity and so it is logical that it may well be linked. Whatever the cause, many children report marked improvements in this respect during the programme.

Poor social skills or lack of sensitivity to other people often causes folk to be regarded as slightly eccentric or odd. In extreme cases, it is called Asperger's Syndrome and it is also a feature of autistic spectrum disorder (ASD), but is often experienced in a mild form by many with learning difficulties. It could well be that, when communication (listening and speaking) is impaired by lack of automaticity in verbal and auditory processing, so much of the brain processing capacity is already in use, thus, the ability to also take in and process (at the same time) observation of those subtleties in body language is limited and, consequently, their social skills are severely constrained. You can guess the benefits of expanding this capacity for such people. It increases their ability to learn or automatise how to react appropriately in social situations and also to read and understand social cues at the same time as they are processing what they want to say. Giving this skill to young children often means they have the chance to develop proper friendships for the first time and also to show affection more readily. For older patients, it usually means improved social awareness and sensitivity to the feelings of others, leaving them feeling more confident in social situations.

Problems showing affection or empathy are similar in origin. Again, in the extreme cases, this is called Asperger's Syndrome or ASD and it can also be explained by limitations in the processing capacity of working memory. People with these symptoms have to work much harder than others in carrying out everyday tasks for themselves, and have little 'spare' capacity to enable them to

work out what the needs of others are so they can be empathetic. In Susie's case, it has been thrilling to watch her move from being in a sort of 'survival' mode to becoming a woman who now has a greater ability to care about how others are feeling.

Maintaining eye contact is quite a problem for some too. When their brains are working hard on listening and speaking, it seems they are unable to process the control of their eyes at the same time and they fail to focus on the person to whom they are talking. This can result in children being judged as 'odd' or 'rude' and in adults this trait is often interpreted as (quite unfairly) an indication that they are dishonest or insincere. Once again, our findings show that it is impossible for the individual to act otherwise, but by resolving the underlying physiological problem, they often seem to find that eye contact is easier to maintain.

Poor posture is complained of by some who find they slouch or hang their head low, or on one side, before going through the programme. This may well be due to insufficient or weak sensory information coming from the nervous system to control their posture. Research from Sheffield University shows that weak muscle tone is commonly seen in people with learning issues. Quite commonly, the programme improves posture – we can only at this stage guess why!

Where travel sickness is a current problem, this is frequently reduced and sometimes goes away completely during treatment as it seems the cerebellum's role in co-ordinating balance and the body's reaction to movement is improved.

Poor sleep patterns are a common problem associated with poor learning, particularly in the younger ones, and often improve somewhat during the programme. This is another result we are still not able to explain, but it is frequently reported by parents. For some it means their children start going to sleep at normal

times, while others find they do not need to sleep abnormally late every morning.

These are just some of the symptoms it seems could well be affected by an incomplete development of the cerebellum. As you can see, there is a lot of exciting research that needs to be done to explain the phenomenon we are observing every day in our centres. Of course nobody, not even Susie, displays all of the things referred to above, but we repeatedly discover that many have far more symptoms than they think, but that they had never before realised that they might be limited to one root cause.

LEARNING STYLES

When you think about it, it is obvious that all those children who experience lack of automaticity in eye tracking and also in auditory processing will suffer dreadfully in the classroom. The teaching styles that teachers heavily rely on involve children being able to listen and pay attention and also to read. Thus, the child who has benefited from the cerebellar development programme will find that they react positively to a broader range of learning styles, especially those in the classroom.

Chapter 8

HOW DOES THIS EXERCISE PROGRAMME WORK?

Through our research, we noticed that people diagnosed with ADHD or dyslexia found reading tiring and difficult, and admitted that they often 'jumped' words and missed them out altogether. A few of those with most of the other common symptoms said they could actually read reasonably well. However, many were not, in fact, 'reading' in the normal sense of the word at all but were using their photographic memory of the shapes of words to attempt to recognise them. Often they would jump from word to word, occasionally missing one, and guessing what should be in the gaps. Many found that, having read a paragraph, often they had not completely taken it in and so had to read it again.

Using the neurological measuring devices and computer analysis that we had developed, it soon became clear that there was a common feature amongst dyslexics and ADHD sufferers. Remarkably, most of them had not completely developed skills in co-ordinating some of their movements and balance. We had

worked out that dyslexics have problems reading because their eyes jump about, as they do not automatically follow the words along the line.

Later, we made the connection between other symptoms and similar traits of incomplete neurological development. Using these results and the latest research evidence, we were able to deduce that poor cerebellar development can be caused by problems in the links between the 'vestibular' (part of the balance mechanism of the inner ear) and the cerebellum itself. It was undeniable that, on average, those people with symptoms of learning difficulties were performing far worse than average in tests designed to measure vestibular input into the cerebellum.

We found that in affected people:

- The cerebellum had not developed as quickly as other parts of the brain and body
- They were often very clever, but underachieving academically
- Frequently, they were exhausted at the end of the day because of the huge amounts of effort they needed to carry out everyday tasks compared to their peers
- Doing everyday things often felt like 'jogging through syrup'.

Our discoveries about the cerebellum made us realise that many experts who deal with learning difficulties were focusing on only part of the problem. Generally, schools only have the resources to tackle a few of the symptoms of learning difficulties, like reading and language skills. While helping these issues is, of course, vitally important in assisting dyslexics and those suffering with

ADHD to develop coping strategies, these techniques are unlikely to resolve the underlying root cause of the problems.

Recent research shows that some of the most common drugs used to help with ADHD are, in fact, targeting the same areas in the cerebellum where we now believe the underdevelopment lies. The drugs appear to be working by 'supercharging' the underdeveloped cerebellum and temporarily allowing it to function as if it is more fully developed. A significant proportion of those who have been prescribed drugs would prefer not to take them because of the concern about possible side-effects. Many, who have been using a drug-based treatment, report that after being on the Dore Programme for a while they are able to come off the prescribed drugs and never need to use them again. We are currently undertaking a research project so that we can provide more guidance to help the large numbers taking prescription medication to be successfully weaned off them, while gaining all the benefits that this new exercise programme brings them.

Some recommend the use of long-chain fatty acid supplements and other nutrients. These products also seem to have a limited effect in increasing the capacity of an underdeveloped cerebellum. Nevertheless, it seems likely there is no retained physiological benefit once they stop taking the supplements.

In recent years, quite a number of children have been prescribed coloured lenses to assist with reading and some report they find them beneficial. What may be happening is that, when these lenses are used, their filtering effect means there is a reduction in the 'amount of data' that has to be processed by the cerebellum (there are fewer wavelengths to process). A brain suffering from processing-capacity problems is more able to cope with this reduced level of information flow. While it does seem to

help the reading symptoms with some of those who try them, it is, of course, dealing with the symptom rather than the root cause. So if, we concluded, the underlying cause of ADHD and dyslexia, and other learning difficulties is incomplete cerebellar development, then we must find a way of forcing that development to take place.

We knew two things. First, the drugs often prescribed to help these symptoms seem to have much of their impact in the cerebellum. This encouraged us that we were targeting the right area, which was further supported by the results of a very recent fMRI study. fMRI stands for functional Magnetic Resonance Imaging – in effect taking pictures of the brain 'when it is functioning'. This particular study, which took place at the world famous University of London centre for brain imaging in Queens Square, indicated that the density of grey matter in a specific area of the cerebellum has a link to reading ability. Second, we knew that by carrying out certain targeted co-ordination exercises it forced the development of new neural pathways in a specific part of the cerebellum. In other words, very targeted, specific repetitious exercises could be used to stimulate and develop these areas of the cerebellum.

Therefore, we developed powerful software to determine the appropriate exercises that would help progressively continue the development precisely where needed. In themselves, these exercises look easy enough, but they are, in fact, very carefully chosen specifically for that individual to match the developmental needs of their cerebellum. They are designed to develop it carefully and systematically over the period of a few months in order that it can acquire the essential capability that enables them to learn and automatise the various types of knowledge and skills that we store in our brain.

Many people have asked me why we cannot create a set of generic exercises that can be used to treat all people with learning difficulties. The truth is that no two people are wired exactly the same way. While it would be extremely useful and efficient to put groups in a room and have a situation like an aerobics lesson in a gym with everyone simultaneously doing the same exercises, it is unlikely to bring out anything like the full potential of everybody in the group. What's worse is that those with the most significant problems would probably benefit least; the exact opposite of what you want.

It is worth remembering that the cerebellum is a phenomenal mass of neural pathways, like little motorways, streets and lanes. All of these neural roads help link everything up and allow the process of learning, or automatising, to take place properly, naturally and normally. Because the cerebellum is such a complicated organ, it is not easy to detect which neural pathways need to be developed. Each individual displays a unique set of characteristics or symptoms.

It is a cliché but the fact is we are all unique; we have unique personalities as we are all wired differently and, therefore, we all have different needs. We doubt if anyone will ever find a generic programme that works really well for all people with learning difficulties. Thus, each of our clients has their own uniquely tuned programme, which corresponds to their needs and corrects the specific areas in the brain where they do not have enough density of neural pathways.

Once it has been determined that a new client is likely to benefit from this programme, they are given a set of specifically selected exercises that are easy and fun to do. These must be carried out twice a day at home (although a few schools now make arrangements for children on the programme). As some do

not find routines easy, we provide clear instruction leaflets and a calendar explaining how and when the exercises must be done.

SO WHAT ARE THESE EXERCISES?

The nature of these exercises varies from person to person, depending on the area of the cerebellum in need of work and the degree of sensory stimulation appropriate. However, generally they start off being pretty easy and become more challenging as progress is made through the programme. However, each has been designed to stimulate at the right level by conducting certain tasks, which are usually a specific combination of co-ordination activities. To be effective, they must be done in the right order and for a prescribed length of time. Here are some examples of just how simple some of the exercises are:

- Throwing a beanbag from hand to hand, following its movement with your eyes, but keeping your head still
- Hopping on one leg in a large circle, first clockwise then anticlockwise, then doing the same on the other leg
- Sitting upright on a chair, turning the head from side to side, pausing only to focus on a chosen point.

Exercises like these and many, many more have been designed to develop in a systematic way the neural pathways that improve balance, hand-to-eye co-ordination and eye tracking, as well as many other aspects of cerebellar function. In the course of a programme, you will do scores of different exercises, all selected to help drive the continued development of the cerebellum and, as you progress to increasingly difficult exercises, you should see how much you are improving at the exercises themselves as well as in your daily life.

On their own the exercises are almost too simple to believe, but they are systematically stimulating the nerve pathways linking the vestibular (inner ear), the cerebrum (thinking brain) and the cerebellum (hindbrain), which then automatises and co-ordinates the memory, emotions, the senses, muscles and the eyes. The programme is carefully formulated to develop the neural pathways progressively, simulating as closely as possible the way they should have developed naturally in early life. The neurological tests are repeated throughout the programme at six-weekly intervals to monitor and determine how the development is progressing, so that the exercises you are given can be adjusted to take the development to the next stage.

Once the targeted part of the cerebellum has developed fully, learning the type of skill that specific part of the cerebellum is responsible for becomes much easier. It seems that when we develop new neural pathways, these create permanent skills that we will never lose – rather like riding a bicycle! In people who have completed the programme, we have not seen any sign of regression in those new skills. In fact, most report they continue to experience even more improvements well after the programme has been completed! In a recent school study, the children made virtually as much academic progress in the year after the programme as the year spent doing the programme. They continue to make more progress than the children in that school who never had a problem. In fact, their academic levels are generally in line with national averages; just a little 'poke in the eye' for those who thought it was a 'placebo effect'.

Over 90 per cent of the people who have completed our programme show substantial improvements in their balance and co-ordination (vestibular performance). This affects their memory,

their emotions, their eye movements and speech. The result is usually a leap in their ability to read, write and lead happier lives. Unprompted, teachers often comment that kids participate more in class; their posture improves; they want to join in team games; they make more friends and start to join in.

THE PROGRAMME: A STEP-BY-STEP GUIDE

'I was worried about visiting the centre. I thought it would be like going to the doctor but they had loads of toys and the people were very friendly.'

Bradley, nine

'It is a bright smiley place and they made us feel right at home. We look forward to our visits now!'

Maggie, Bradley's mum

Before someone starts an exercise programme like this, it is necessary to make sure that it is the development (or lack of development) of the cerebellum that is causing the problem. In virtually all cases that come to us, we find that it is, but of course that is not always the case. Therefore, a therapist should spend time building up a detailed picture of each person before they begin the programme.

GOING THROUGH A PROGRAMME

In a typical centre there would be a wide range of highly trained people who understand all the main issues of learning and behavioural problems. With the input from these specialists who conduct detailed assessments and several neurological tests, a profile of the way in which the individual currently performs certain key tasks of mental and physical co-ordination is built up.

This is done for two reasons: first, it allows the computer software to put together exactly the combination of exercises needed to develop the specific area of the cerebellum. Second, it means there are a number of baseline measures to keep a close and accurate track of progress at each subsequent visit.

THE OCULOMOTOR OR 'EYE-TRACKING' TESTS

These tests (called the oculomotor or OMT test, which measures the accuracy of eye tracking) are done to show exactly how the eye is moving when it is tracking a moving object. They involve sitting still in a darkened room (a parent will always accompany a child) with a specialist operating the equipment. Sticky pads holding electrodes are attached to the head to measure muscle response and record how the eye is moving. The person is then asked to follow a red light moving from side to side, moving only their eyes and keeping their head still. Sometimes the light moves randomly, sometimes alternating left and right at varying speeds, other times in a rapid succession to one side or the other. The whole process takes about half an hour and the results are plotted on a computer printout that clearly shows the actual movements relative to the desired track.

Since eye tracking is a crucial guide to the activity of the cerebellum, and gives an indication of fine motor skills, it can show very clearly if there are any development problems. When the test is repeated at subsequent visits, it usually shows the eye tracking is improving. Very often, this amazes folk, who see clearly for the very first time why they have had such difficulties with reading. They then ask, 'I have had this problem my whole life, so why on earth has nobody shown me this before?'

THE POSTUROGRAPHY (OR BALANCE STRATEGY TEST)

In some ways, this is the most important test and, because it provides so much information, it usually needs to be repeated every visit throughout the exercise programme. The measurements it provides (worked out using sophisticated computer software) show how the cerebellum copes with controlling posture and balance, and helps determine which areas of the cerebellum need to be developed. This information allows the selection and prescription of the specific exercises that will help that individual most effectively.

Many people with learning difficulties are particularly good at using the senses they feel through the joints and muscles of the body (called 'somatosensory' feelings). This is because in this group of people vestibular or 'inner-ear' senses that normally help with balance are largely ignored by the cerebellum. In our experience, we have found that in almost every such case their brain uses their vestibular senses far less than they should, but, as the development programme progresses, this is steadily corrected.

During the balance strategy test, patients stand on a platform with moveable footplates. They will be asked to maintain their balance while a whole series of tests are done: first, with their eyes open and then closed, sometimes with everything stationary, other times with the footplates moving. The way their body responds is fed into the computer that calculates how the cerebellum uses the various sensory inputs. It reveals balance problems and speed of response to change of movement. Some can find this somewhat difficult initially, particularly when asked to do it with their eyes shut. However, as the exercise programme takes effect, those same people enjoy seeing how much their ability to perform these tests improves with each visit.

SPECIALISED MEMORY-PROCESSING TESTS

It is normal to use a large range of verbal, computer and written tests developed to assess how people cope with processing words and numbers. Some of these are likely to include actions such as threading beads and using a computer mouse to track movements on the screen. This also gives a good indication of how well developed their fine motor skills are, and the results are fed into the software to help form the prescription of an exercise programme.

TALKING IT OVER

Once the results of all the tests have been processed, the person will sit down with a doctor or other specialist, and talk through the way in which this information helps us determine the root cause of their symptoms. This is a process most seem to appreciate. It can be an emotional moment when you feel the relief of knowing that you are not 'thick' and there is a physiological explanation for all the frustrations and problems you have experienced.

THE EXERCISE PROGRAMME

If appropriate for the programme, they will then be given the specifically selected exercises. These must be carried out twice each day, usually at home (although a few schools now make arrangements for children on the programme). Many do not find routines easy, so it is necessary to provide clear instruction leaflets and a calendar explaining how and when the exercises must be done. Some simple equipment will normally be required – beanbags, wobble boards (plastic, circular discs, about 1ft in diameter. The discs have a semi-circular attachment on the underside that lift them approximately 2 inches from the ground.

When a person stands on them, it forces their balance organs to work harder), exercise balls and eye exercise charts.

WHAT HAPPENS NEXT?

Patients need to return to be retested at six-week intervals to check up on progress and so they can see their results graphically and, as their various functions improve, have their exercise programme amended accordingly. To be able to see improvement in the cerebellar function right in front of your eyes is wonderfully encouraging!

FINISHING THE PROGRAMME

Once a person has successfully completed the whole programme, it would be usual for cerebellar function to be in the 'normal range' for people their age. Simply, this means their brain now functions in a normal and typical way: their handicap to learning or automatising has been eradicated as far as possible and they haven't been taught anything. However, what has happened is that they are now more able to learn, to remember things and to recall that information when they need it. Certainly, this makes life easier for their teachers. But, most importantly, it is the life of the individual that should improve in a way they would never before have imagined possible.

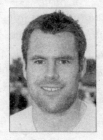

KENNY LOGAN?S STORY

'Outside of having twins the programme was the best thing I have ever done. I have played for my country and done lots of other amazing things, but I am more excited about my life now than ever before.'

For years, Scottish rugby star Kenny Logan hid his literacy difficulties behind a mask of bravado. It was only when his wife Gabby told him about the new treatment that he had the courage to tackle his dyslexia.

Living with dyslexia

'Trying to recall the details of what happened during my school life is really difficult for me. I was not a happy child and I spent the majority of the time just trying to keep my head down. As soon as I left school all my memories suddenly become much more clear and vivid, but before that it is all a bit of a blur. It is hard to sit here now and remember specific details about what I went through. Rather, when I think back to that time, I am overwhelmed with a sense of sadness about missed opportunities and a wasted life.

'All through high school I was called "stupid" or "thick" by teachers and other pupils. The main reason for this was that I couldn't read or write. I had never managed to get my head around the alphabet, or understand why certain combinations of letters made certain sounds.

I couldn't understand why words like "phone" were not spelled "fone", and the more I tried to understand it, the more confused I got. It was as if there was a six-year-old boy inside me, who was trapped and couldn't grow up. I wanted so desperately to catch up with everyone else and I sometimes would cry myself to sleep.

'In the end I spent most of my school life trying to get myself kicked out of the classroom. I felt more comfortable standing out in the corridor than sitting in an environment where I could be picked on. I used to do all sorts of stupid things to get myself thrown out, like hiding behind the blackboard or passing notes. I was not a bully at school or an attention seeker, but I did act up in certain classes where I felt threatened. I simply got fed up of being made to feel stupid and preferred to be in a place where I would not be noticed.

'Quite often, I would miss classes because I was ill – well, I thought I was ill but in actual fact I used to get terrible stomach pains because I was so nervous and worried about school. These pains seemed to get worse as I went through school. There is no doubt in my mind that these pains were brought on by worry and nervousness. I remember waking up every morning with a panicky feeling in my stomach, as if someone was about to punch me. The closer I got to school, the more tension I would feel until sometimes the pain would be excruciating.

'Every single day I would try and self-motivate myself by saying, "I am going to try my hardest today!" but, no matter what I did, things did not get any better. Somehow,

I always ended up getting told off for making mistakes. There just did not seem to be that level of understanding amongst teachers that there is today. Nobody seemed to realise that I needed help and they just assumed I was being lazy.

'In the end the only thing that got me through school was sport. I loved rugby, football, golf and anything where I could be active. Being a farmer's son, there was something about being outside that felt so natural to me. Running around the playing field was fun and enjoyable, and so much better than being in a stuffy classroom. The physical pain I would feel from being knocked to the ground in rugby was nothing compared to the mental pain I would feel when I was trying to read. I also liked the fact that, if I did well in rugby, I'd get patted on the back and hear people say, "Well done, Kenny!"

'When it came to doing my GCSEs, however, I was not so confident. As I sat down to take my first exam and opened the paper, the first thing that went through my mind was that I couldn't read the questions. I spent five minutes trying to make sense of the words, but the harder I tried, the more confused I became. I sat back in my chair and glanced around at my classmates with their heads down scribbling and realised I couldn't do this. I stood up and walked out of the exam, vowing that I would never come back. That was the end of my education and without any qualifications I left school at 16.

'I worked on a farm from the ages of 16 to 24. During

this time, I had started playing rugby professionally and I was capped for Scotland when I was 19. Playing rugby for my country was something I had wanted to do my whole life. I clearly remember being nine and kicking a rugby ball on my farm for the first time. At that moment, I knew that I wanted to be a rugby player.

'But even when I became a professional rugby player I still felt like a six-year-old child inside. When I went down to play for Wasps in 1996, I did not think about the fact that I was going to be playing for the best team in Europe, I was more worried about how I was going to cope living alone in London where nobody knew me. I still couldn't read or write, and I couldn't even write my new London address. I was being sent hundreds of forms through my letterbox every day and I did not know what to do. In the end, I had to send them back home to my mum for her to deal with them for me. I am glad she did because otherwise I wouldn't have been able to pay my bills.

'The real embarrassment came when I would be travelling around with Wasps and I had to fill in forms and applications. When the coach sat down with me one day and asked me to complete a fitness form, I went into a panic. I was 24 years old and it was beyond me. I had to tell him I was dyslexic and that I couldn't do it. It was the first time I'd told anybody, other than close family, about my problem and I was a bit anxious about how he would react. Thankfully, he was pretty cool about the whole thing and he got a fitness guy to go through everything with me and fill the form in.

'With someone helping to fill in forms and with my mum still helping me when I needed to write things out, I thought I might just be able to get through life without dyslexia being an issue. It was not really until I started going out with Gabby, when I was 27, that I started to think about it again.

'One day, after we had just started going out, Gabby was reading an article that had been written about her when she turned to me and asked what I thought about it. I looked at the page for about five minutes and I replied I thought it was really good. She looked surprised and said she was amazed how quickly I had managed to read the article. I tried to shrug the whole thing off and told her I had always been a quick reader. Gabby then looked me in the eye and said, "You're dyslexic, aren't you?"

'Over the next few years, Gabby kept bringing up the fact that I was dyslexic. She would say things like, "In the past whenever someone has said something against you, you've always proved them wrong. Whenever someone has said you couldn't deliver, you've gone ahead and done it. Yet your whole life you've been running away from dyslexia." I knew she was right, but I didn't know what I was supposed to do about it. I wanted to beat it, but I didn't know how.

'I used to be scared about my future. After all, you cannot play rugby until you're 60 and I didn't know what I was going to do after I had finished.

'I was about 30 when Tonight with Trevor McDonald broadcast. Gabby and I videoed it and watched it together.

I couldn't believe what I was seeing. The Dore Programme sounded amazing; it sounded too good to be true. I could relate to every person in the documentary. They all seemed to share my story and I even cried a bit. It made me think about all the things I'd never been able to do. For example, I couldn't sit on a beach on holiday and read a book. Gabby would get through about five a week and I could barely get through five pages. With Gabby's full support, I decided to give the programme a go.

'As soon as I walked into the Dore Centre in Fulham, I started to feel uneasy about the whole thing. I was 30 years old, I had 55 caps for my country, and here I was sitting in a room with a six-year-old, an eight-year-old and a 14-year-old. All of them were nervous, but none more so than me. I kept thinking, What if they ask me a question and I can't answer it? I was a grown man and I was terrified of embarrassing myself.

'I was relieved to find that the test they gave me was very relaxed. I was asked to spell different words, which got progressively harder. The staff were really warm and friendly, and put me at ease straight away.

'After they had diagnosed me, I was prescribed a set of exercises to do every day. The exercises included things like throwing a beanbag from one hand to the other. They were so simple and straightforward that I was a bit doubtful about them at first. I kept thinking, What is this doing for me?

'I went back every six weeks for retests and each time I was prescribed a different set of exercises. The exercises got harder and harder. For example, there was one exercise

where I had to spin around ten times, stop and then spin in the other direction. I could only do a few of these before I would feel violently sick.'

The changes
'After a few months of doing the exercises I started to notice some changes. The staff at the clinic had warned me that, while my neural pathways built up to improve my co-ordination, I might start to get a bit clumsy. They said I might start dropping things and notice other differences while my balance was readjusting. Yet, even with this advice, I was not prepared for what happened.

'At rugby practice I started to have problems holding on to the balls. I was dropping them all the time and in the end the coach had to come up to me to check I was all right. I remember thinking that if I kept this up I would get sacked. I remember once playing against Bath. I caught the ball and ran straight into touch. There was an opposition player in sight. I could see people were looking at me completely baffled. As I looked down and saw the line, I was just as confused as everyone else was – it was as if someone had actually moved it when I wasn't looking.

'My co-ordination was getting so bad that I was seriously considering dropping off the programme. After all, as much as I wanted to beat dyslexia, I did not want to get fired over it. I went back to the clinic and they told me that I had really responded well and that, if I was able to hold on for another few weeks, I would find things would get better.

'I am glad I listened to their advice and stuck at it because that season was to turn into one of the best seasons I had ever had for Scotland and for Wasps. It was not long before I'd regained balance and co-ordination and I stopped dropping balls. I was greatly relieved by this and I was also surprised to notice my game had actually improved. I found I was able to concentrate for the full 80 minutes and was constantly making the right decisions. Before I'd done the programme, I'd had tunnel vision. I'd been a good solid player, but I had always been single-minded and focused on the things going on in front of me. Suddenly, it was as if someone had suddenly switched on a light and I was able to see everything that was going on around me.

'A few months later, Scotland were playing in the 2003 World Cup. Even though I'd now been on the programme for a long time, dyslexia was still something I was embarrassed about. I couldn't even tell the Scotland captain, Brian Redpath, who was one of my best mates. When the other guys were going for breakfast, I would pop back to my room and do some exercises. Sometimes I would pretend I'd forgotten something in the hotel and use that as an excuse to get a session done then.

'There were a number of times when I felt like skipping an exercise session, but I just kept reminding myself about the results I'd seen. This was a programme where there had been a 95 per cent success rate. The chances that I would be among those 5 per cent who it did not work for were pretty slim so I knew I had to keep rigorously to the schedule. In the end, the results proved I had been right to

do this. It was not just my rugby game that was flying; there had been all sorts of changes taking place that other people were starting to notice.

'I started to pick things up quicker and say things that were more relevant to conversations. These were subtle changes but they did not go unnoticed. For example, after games we would be talking about our performance and I would point out mistakes and explain why those mistakes were made, and make suggestions for improvements. This was something I'd never done before.

'Gradually, I began to notice more and more improvements. The Dore Clinic had always described the brain as a library and the cerebellum as a librarian. It was as if all my life my own library had been completely messed up, with books lying all over the place. Now, though, my librarian was beginning to do his job and had started putting things in order. One night, when I was lying in bed, I started to think about the times tables, which I had always had problems with. As I concentrated harder and harder, it was as if everything just fell into place; it suddenly made sense. I couldn't get to sleep that night because equations kept forming in my head. The more I thought about it, the more I understood it.

'My spelling also improved dramatically. I remember once asking Gabby how to spell Belfast. She spelled it out for me: "B.E.L.F.A.S.T." The next day when I had to write that word I actually remembered the spelling. Before doing the programme, I would have had to ask Gabby that spelling every day for the rest of my life.

'A few years later, when I was with a group of other Dore graduates, I spelled out the word "cerebellum". I had only seen the word a few times before, but the letters just formed in my mind without any trouble. I'd never done anything like that before and I was more excited about it than anything. Wynford Dore was at the meeting and I saw him looking at me with his mouth wide open.

'I can write cheques now. Before I would make excuses like I'd hurt my hand. I can also read books and I am a big fan of autobiographies and other non-fiction books. My confidence has also grown as a result of the programme. Public speaking is something I would never have done before. It is much easier to stand in front of a TV camera than stand up and speak in front of 500 people. But now I can easily get up in front of an audience and tell them about how the programme has changed my life; I even enjoy it.

'In short, the programme is something I completely believe in. It changed my whole life and every day I hear stories about how it changed other people's lives. I am not going to say my spelling and reading are 100 per cent perfect, but I have been given the foundation to build upon. To make the best of this, I have started to have a personal tutor to help fill in the gaps I missed when I was at school. It is so great to know that, this time around, I am actually learning something.

'What the programme has really given me is a second chance at life. My sport used to overshadow my life and I was worried that one day I would look back and say my best years were when I played rugby. Now I am far more

excited about my future than I am about my past. I set up a company, Logan Group, six years ago responsible for events and sponsorship. I was really proud of the venture, but I realised that, unless I was able to move on, the company would not be able to move on. Now I am so much more organised and aware of things, and the company is going from strength to strength.

'I really hope that Wynford is able to achieve his ambition and make the programme available to everyone. We need to give kids an opportunity to learn so that they may go and do what they want to do. If someone who can read and write wants to be a bricky or a labourer, then they should be allowed to go and do that. In the same way, if someone wants to be a doctor, they should be given the opportunity to learn so they can get on with it.'

Thank you, Wynford.

Chapter 9

HOW THE MEDIA HELPED

Media interest in what we were doing grew at an alarming rate, so much so that I had to employ a media professional, Nigel Robinson, to help me communicate with and then select those with whom we would spend time communicating. Whatever we did seemed to create a media frenzy. I'll never forget doing 13 TV and radio interviews in one day in January 2001. At the end of my last interview that day, I was asked to appear on yet another programme, the *Johnny Walker Drive Time Show*. I was so exhausted I did not want to go, but eventually succumbed to persuasion. By the time I arrived at the BBC studio, I was having real trouble keeping my eyes open. Before going on air, they gave me a briefing sheet to read, but the page was just a blur and I couldn't take it in.

When I finally sat down, I was relieved to find Johnny Walker to be a delightful personality. After asking me a couple of questions, he let me go into 'transmit mode', and I went on for about 20 minutes. During this time, I hardly stopped for breath. I was running on autopilot and was just trying to get my message out as succinctly as

I could. I poured my heart out about how desperate the problem was, how many parents and teachers were so concerned, and how wonderful and effective this new remediation process seemed to be.

At the end of that transmission, I went and slept in the back of the car for the entire journey home. For weeks, the phones at our offices in Kenilworth were in meltdown. People who had heard the Johnny Walker show were calling in to talk about how their children had exactly the same symptoms as Susie. Many of these people, without hesitation, did the programme and, as a result, our centre was busy for several months, purely on the back of that one single broadcast. Little did I realise that this would be a small drop in the ocean compared to the impact that a single TV documentary was going to have!

Not long after our first centre opened, we were approached by more than a dozen filmmakers wanting to make documentaries about this 'new breakthrough'. It would have been wonderful to have had several people making programmes about the treatment, but in the end I had to choose to work with only one. The obvious choice was ITV's *Tonight with Trevor McDonald*, which reached by far the biggest audience (about 2.8 million people) and was one of the most talked-about news programmes in Britain at the time.

The producer, Susanne Rock, was very keen for the programme to follow a group of people going through the programme. She wanted to interview them about their whole experience of suffering with learning difficulties. This was a refreshing and exciting approach – if we did not simply provide the film-makers with people to be interviewed, but allowed them to film openly with some of those taking part, viewers seeing the extent of the changes would have no reason to fear there had been some sort of set-up. I wanted the documentary to be gripping and

convincing. The only way to do this was to put the whole treatment in the spotlight and test it publicly. After talking it over with Susanne, who was an awesome filmmaker and taught me so much, we agreed on a simple approach: ITV independently found and selected people to go through the programme. I was confident enough that the treatment would work. This was prime-time national TV, a huge platform from which to show people the true possibilities, and I knew I could not waste the opportunity. In no time at all, several candidates had been chosen. They all suffered from learning or attention symptoms and were all in need of help.

I was immensely grateful that all of these prospective patients were prepared to carry out the exercises diligently over a period of time. I knew that it did not matter whether they believed in the treatment or not, the only thing that mattered was that they did the exercises every day. If they did not perform their daily routine then it wouldn't work. Thankfully, this was an issue we never had to face – the patients were all honest, good people, and they did what was asked of them. It was not long before we started to see changes taking place across the board and by the end of the course they couldn't believe the changes that were happening for them.

Knowing that the documentary was shaping up to be a success, I began to seriously think about the implications of the broadcast being viewed by an audience of 3 million people. Given the impact of the Johnny Walker interview, we were likely to be swamped with interest. Abruptly, all the issues of scaling up the fledgling operation hit me in a way like never before.

As time ticked away and the date of the broadcast (21 January 2002) became closer and closer, we were forced to make decisions in a fast, furious and remarkably unstructured way. One classic instance of this was the manner in which we decided to open our eighth centre. In addition to Kenilworth, we had

originally planned to open six new centres that were to be located in London, Cardiff, Bedford, Manchester, Sheffield and Edinburgh. By mistake, however, one of our staff told the press that we were speculating about opening an eighth centre in Southampton. They reported this and, because of all the exposure, we decided we had to roll with it. Within two weeks, we had found the staff and then suitable premises near by soon after, and we were in a position to open in Southampton as well.

As you can imagine, I was pulling in favours from every friend and acquaintance I had. Everything was happening so fast it was an absolute blur. Thankfully, luck and serendipity were on my side and the whole project continued to zoom forward at breakneck speed. There seemed to be a lot of luck involved – for instance, I obtained premises in Manchester from a landlord at a very favourable rate. This was solely down to the fact that the landlord had a son who had gone through our programme. He wanted to do all he could to help Dore Centres open in this area. This was a classic example of the sort of unexpected help I suddenly found myself receiving from many quarters.

With everything delicately poised, I now waited with a sickening sense of anticipation for the Trevor McDonald programme to be broadcast. I had prepared the ground as much as I could by finding premises and advertising for staff. However, I had stopped short of actually employing the huge extra numbers needed, or signing any contracts until the documentary went to air and, as I hoped would happen, the phones started to ring.

With the medium-term future of the organisation in the balance, I waited on tenterhooks.

21 JANUARY 2002

My mobile phone only works in certain rooms in my house. In

some rooms, the walls are three feet thick and not even the most powerful handset can pick up a reception. Just an hour or so before the Trevor McDonald programme went to air, I randomly walked into one of the rooms where my phone does happen to work, and it started to ring. On the other line was the producer, who sounded frantic. She was desperate to get the answer to a last-minute technical query prior to the show being aired. I gave her the appropriate answer and that was that. It was only later that I discovered that, if I had not answered my phone, the producers would have been stuck on an important last-minute check and might have had to re-edit some of the film, working against the clock – and that could have changed absolutely everything.

What proceeded from the airing of the documentary was the most amazing sequence of events. Thanks to the Johnny Walker experience, we had anticipated that there would be a significant number of phone calls. So, we had employed the use of a call centre in Glasgow that had some 150 operators working on the phones. What I had not anticipated was that many people with learning difficulties often write numbers down in the wrong sequence. As a result, many people trying to call us kept dialling incorrect numbers.

Consequently, that evening the British Telecom directory enquiries service was so overloaded with calls that it crashed. British Telecom's Glasgow Exchange also crashed that evening, such was the demand. In fact, for the following two months we had to use our mobile phones to make any outgoing calls at all!

By the time morning arrived, we were incredibly relieved that we had prepared the ground to open eight new centres throughout the UK. Many people had driven their cars from various parts of the country overnight and had parked outside the clinic in Kenilworth to ensure they would be the first to book appointments. As we had already interviewed the staff, negotiated all the leases and

manufactured the equipment, we were able to press all the green buttons and very quickly everything was in motion. Within 12 weeks, we had some 150 new staff treating thousands of children and adults, who had been signed up as a result of the broadcast.

In fact, from June 2001 to March 2002, our operation increased twenty-fold in staff. Thanks to our new software, we were able to train therapists from a number of backgrounds, particularly nursing and teaching, so that was not a constraint. The key attribute that we were looking for was good patient communication skills; the software we had developed would deal with the more technical aspects of the job automatically.

Despite the fast-paced nature of our recruitment, we were very fortunate to end up with a team with an enormous amount of initiative and determination. A large proportion of those who joined us at that time had family members who had suffered from learning difficulties. They were well versed in the heartache of the condition and were very passionate about our cause. It was quite clear that they all got it! They understood what we were trying to do and wanted to be involved in any way they could.

Watching it all happen filled me with an overpowering sense of pride in my wonderful team, not to mention relief. While my role had been to co-ordinate and put everything together, the programme would not have become a reality without each and every one of so many key people. Every one of them was vital and, looking back, it is clear that, had they not been at the right place at the right time, this whole project could have failed.

The clear consequence of the awareness created by the media is that we had the chance to help thousands of people quickly while at the same time collecting large quantities of valuable research data to measure and demonstrate the remarkable effectiveness of what had been developed.

Chapter 10

BALSALL COMMON SCHOOL – FIRST RESEARCH PROJECT

'In my 22-year career as a headmaster I have never witnessed a programme which has had such a great impact on children's learning.'

Trevor Davies, headmaster of Balsall Common Primary School

The success of the venture and the feedback from people who attended our centres took us happily by surprise. We seemed to have unlocked a simple, but tremendously important solution to a problem that is debilitating for an enormous number of people. To cope with the huge demand from people wanting to join, we quickly had to expand the service. By early 2005, over 18,000 people – children and adults – had enrolled on the programme.

In 2001–03, two professors undertook an independent research initiative in a large primary school near Coventry, which, on the face of it, had a perfectly normal proportion of children with learning difficulties. The reason for this was to provide an independent measure of the effectiveness of the treatment.

TREVOR DAVIES

One day, I received a phone call from the headmaster of a local school. He had been watching the news coverage of our programme and wanted to know more. We invited him down to our centre and it turned out that, not only was he headmaster of Balsall Common Primary School, but he was also a government inspector of schools in the UK. He said he wanted to take a serious look at the things we were doing. His name was Trevor Davies and he was about to help write one of the most important chapters in our history.

Trevor was typical of that wonderful breed of headmaster who cares passionately about their pupils and wants to bring out the best in each and every one them. Already his school had a well-established reputation for taking a very proactive and highly regarded approach to learning difficulties. The existing learning difficulties programme included a high level of special needs support and, if needed, used phonological intervention programmes (a method of teaching reading based on the sounds within each word). Despite this, Trevor told me he was deeply frustrated by the lack of progress made by some of his students.

The first thing he wanted us to do was carry out a 'pilot study'. For this, he would select a pupil to be treated and would observe him firsthand to see if there were any changes. He said that if the experiment was a success we might be allowed to embark upon a much broader research project in his school.

Trevor selected Simon Coleman, the son of some very caring and concerned parents. They were anxious for their son to get into Solihull School, which was the best school in the area, but knew that with his current rate of academic progress this was simply not going to happen.

As you may have guessed, the programme was a complete success with Simon. Now, five years on, he is doing wonderfully well in most subjects. It was amazing to think that just a few years earlier he had been frustrated and falling behind his peers. Trevor was ecstatic about what he was seeing from this pilot study and was happy for us to carry out a full research study in his school, providing of course that we had the support of the parents.

SELECTING THE CANDIDATES

This was our first major research project, which meant we had a big challenge on our hands trying to convince parents to put their children on a new-fangled programme. We were asking them to make their children do a five- to ten-minute exercise session twice a day for up to a year without being able to guarantee that they would see results.

Thankfully, Trevor Davies leaped to our rescue. This was a huge task for him and we were all equally surprised by his endless amounts of determination. Being such a well-respected and trusted figure in the school, he was really putting his reputation on the line for us. He told parents the reasons why he thought the project was a great opportunity, not just for his school but also for schools across the country, who would learn about their experience with the treatment.

Our first task was to identify the children who were not achieving their full potential. We were looking for various signs of possible learning or attention difficulties. Tests used for this study involved a widely used dyslexia screening test (written by the University of Sheffield), DSM IV (attention deficit test), physiological tests (including dynamic posturography) and neurological examinations carried out by a medical doctor. Approximately 20 per cent of the children were identified as

potentially underachieving and we selected a total of 40 candidates for the study.

What was interesting about the whole process was that we soon realised there were many children with learning difficulties who had not been formerly diagnosed as having dyslexia or ADHD. Indeed, of the group we selected, only 30 per cent had been identified and were receiving special-needs support. This gave us one of the first clues that many students who do reasonably well at school could in fact be doing much better still were they not constrained by the incomplete development of their cerebellum.

This observation in itself is fascinating as it highlights how so many students today are able to go right through school without being given any special attention or aid. Balsall Common School had a wonderfully positive attitude towards children with learning issues. There was a great emphasis on openness and support, yet even they had failed to detect a great number of children in need.

It is estimated that there are 5 million people in the UK alone undiagnosed as having learning difficulties that impair them to some extent. The reason for this is that schoolchildren are all too often only identified with a problem either because they are causing disruption in the classroom, or because their results are so poor they are pulling down the statistics of the school. For these students, it is impossible to slip under the mat and, more often than not, they are given extra tuition to try to bring them up to speed. They do not, however, represent the total proportion of the population that would benefit from help. There are millions of exceptionally bright students with learning difficulties who are reasonably able to keep up with the rest of the class. Often, they are the ones who sit quietly and passively

in class and diligently struggle in silence as they desperately work hard not to fall behind. Yet, however hard they study, they are never able to reach their full potential and often have to put at least twice as much effort in as everyone else just to get reasonable grades.

A SCIENTIFIC APPROACH

We realised this research study would be a difficult project to see through and we anticipated there was going to be a lot of criticism, not least from the Establishment, who were, at the time, largely against what we were doing. In order to counter these attacks as best we could, we decided to rely on two top professors to oversee the whole process. We chose Professor Nicolson of Sheffield University, because he was an expert on the cerebellum and cognitive learning processes, and we also selected Professor David Reynolds, formally of Exeter University and now at Plymouth University, because he was widely respected and a very clear thinker. He was the kind of man who was absolutely and only influenced by solid science. Reynolds had been chair of the Numeracy Strategy Committee for the British Department of Education and had sat on the Committee for Literacy Strategy, too. We hoped the combined efforts of these two meticulous researchers would finally and categorically prove whether the treatment was working or not.

One of the first considerations in developing the research programme was the precise design of the study. To my amazement there is no standard way of benchmarking or testing a product or service developed to help us learn, or to help remediate those with learning problems.

Professor Reynolds explained to me that one way to do a scientific study would be to have two groups. One group would

receive the treatment on the programme and the other would receive a placebo treatment (i.e. one that is known to be ineffective). I have to say that I thought this approach was particularly cruel. After all, we were not talking about inanimate objects, but children who only had one chance of going through each year of their school life. I felt that if some of these children missed out the potential benefit for a whole year then this would be of permanent harm to them. If anybody had put Susie on a placebo as part of a trial, I am sure I would have felt inconsolably angry and used. How then could I possibly subject anyone else's child to something I would never have permitted my own children to be part of?

To my simple mind, there was already so much data about children in schools that there was hardly a need to collect more information. The scientists, of course, were arguing that we were giving these children attention, which could be the reason why we were seeing improvements. For me, this did not stand up as a valid argument. If all these patients were experiencing changes simply because we were lavishing them with attention, then there would be no need for the programme at all. If Susie's dramatic transformation was purely as a result of me focusing my attention on her, why hadn't we seen such changes in the past? For years, we had done everything we could to help her, but no amount of attention or concern seemed to make the slightest difference. Finally, she was beginning to move forward and, as far as I was concerned, that had nothing to do with a placebo effect.

The whole control group argument raged on for quite a while. When we asked parents whether they would consider putting their children into a control group, naturally there was quite a hostile reaction. Amongst parents, the feeling was 'if there is a treatment suspected of working, I want my child in that group'. The end conclusion was to use an alternative and, I'm assured,

equally scientific method that involved having a 'changeover' group. One group would start six months before the other. This would help us graph the relative progress of each group and was a method quite acceptable to researchers.

The project, of course, involved the children being tested using our full physiological and neurological tests. They were then given the individual exercises that they were required to carry out at home twice a day.

ANECDOTAL EVIDENCE THAT THE TREATMENT WAS WORKING

In the period of time before the end-of-year results came through, there was so much anecdotal evidence from the school that the programme was working that I was starting to feel more and more relaxed. Trevor Davies told me one day how he had come across a little girl crying in the corridor. She had been discussing her homework with her teacher, who thought that her work had improved so suddenly that she must have cheated. The teacher in question had no idea the little girl was doing the research project because we had wanted to keep it a secret so that the outcome of the experiment would not be affected. All the teacher knew was that normally this student would hand in short, three-line essays for homework and now, suddenly, she was handing in three pages of well-written prose. Quite naturally, she suspected foul play. Thankfully, Trevor had a word with the teacher and straightened everything out.

As similar stories flew in at an increasing rate, our research files were also beginning to bulge under the weight of information. Trevor reported on the progress after six months: '...the results were remarkable – with all of the children making highly significant progress, not only in academic areas such as literacy and numeracy, but also in self-esteem.' He also made

another quite remarkable observation: he noticed that many of those children who had previously shown little interest in sport were becoming involved in school sports teams and showed distinct signs of improvement in motor skills and co-ordination. It was not long before he told me that the school football team was filling up with pupils who had gone through our programme. A few of these budding sports stars had barely been able to kick a ball before the programme and now, suddenly, they were receiving adoration for their skills on the pitch.

It was at this moment that we realised the potential implications our treatment had for sportsmen and women, something we had not dreamed of achieving (for a more detailed explanation of why this is, you may wish to read Chapter 14, pages 199–206). Despite this positive feedback, it seemed, alarmingly, that not quite every child was benefiting from the programme. The parents of two children were adamant that their kids were doing the exercises, but that they were making very little progress academically. After we carried out some neurological tests, however, we had evidence to suggest that this was not quite the case and that actually the students were not performing the exercises every day as required. We confronted the parents outright with this information and finally they admitted that they had not complied with the exercise requirements. It was not long after this meeting that we started to see the first signs of progress in these two students, who were now being made to do the exercises when they should.

Even with a firsthand knowledge of Professor Reynolds's scientific approach, I was still surprised just how clinical and totally unimpressed he was about the things we were seeing. Although he spoke to many parents and witnessed many changes in students over the year, he absolutely refused to say anything

positive about the programme. For him, the only thing he considered worth reacting to would be the final results that would come out at the end of the project.

THE END RESULTS

At the end of phase one of the study, in 2001, the results were analysed and they were stunning; they were way beyond the expectations that we had. Quite often when a gradual and steady change takes place, you do not realise it on a day-by-day basis. For example, it is only when your child puts on an old pair of trousers that rise three inches up their ankle that you can say, 'Wow, you've grown!' For many parents, it must have been a bit like that – suddenly, they realised their child had actually made loads of progress.

After the selected candidates completed the programme, between 2002 and 2003, they took their SATs (Standard Assessment Tests), which all British children take at key stages during their education. The results the professors reported after the programme speak for themselves:

- In comprehension age, the rate of annual improvement increased by almost five times after treatment
- In reading, age the rate of annual improvement increased threefold
- In writing, the rate of annual improvement increased by an extraordinary 17 times
- On top of this, the children's perception of their own happiness, confidence and sporting ability increased in 70 per cent of cases

It was wonderful to see all these changes, but there was one question that dug away at all of us. What we really wanted to

know was, would these improvements last after students had finished the programme? Would they continue to flourish and prosper, or would they regress and still have learning problems? The medial theory was that it should be a permanent solution and now it was time to test our own hope.

A year or so later, after the pupils had finished the course, we tested them again to see whether we had achieved our goal. What followed is once again best summarised by their headmaster Trevor Davies:

> *'While we were delighted with the progress that the pupils taking part in the study made in their first year, we were amazed at the progress they made during their second year of the programme, i.e. the year following the completion of the exercise-based programme. It became evident that we had really made major changes to these pupils' lives. Not only were they on average working at a level appropriate to their age and at the same level as their peers, but some were even exceeding this.'*

Professors Nicolson and Reynolds later published these findings in a paper called 'Evaluation of an Exercise-based Treatment for Children with Learning Difficulties'. They showed that the children with a learning difficulty made greater academic progress than those without learning issues and that, compared to their school peers, the improvements in reading were even better after completing the programme than when they were receiving it.

Professor Reynolds also looked at the mild and more severe dyslexic children and found to his astonishment that the mild dyslexia group showed no signs of dyslexia a year after finishing the programme and that the more severe dyslexia group

improved even more than the mild group, now showing only the slightest indications of still being dyslexic a year after stopping the programme.

In essence, all this meant was that children caught up rapidly with their school peers without receiving any additional teaching support. It showed that we had given them the mental tools they needed to learn and develop and, even though they had by now finished doing the programme, they continued to make strong progress.

What we achieved in Balsall Common is something I'll never forget. Even today, years after we finished the project, there are reminders everywhere. In November 2005, for instance, 13-year-old Lauren Watson, a former pupil from the school, gave a keynote speech at an international conference for all our senior managers from around the world. Lauren had gone through the programme and managed to keep us spellbound for 40 minutes. She told us what her life was like before going through the programme, what life was like during the programme and what it was like afterwards. In addition to this, she told us how she had gone from being quite shy, physically very clumsy and requiring special-needs support to being the youngest instructor in Tae Kwon Do and excelling in her academic subjects.

She spoke to us with a confidence and eloquence that you would not expect from most adults talking at a conference, let alone a 13-year-old child without any notes. Finally, she concluded her talk by pleading with us not to stop our work until we had got our programme into every curriculum of every school, so that every child in need could be helped in the same way as she had been.

Her words had been so poignant and powerful that I found myself overwhelmed with emotion. As I looked around the

conference table, there was not a dry eye in the room. My colleagues and I had been given a vote of confidence by someone who really mattered. As important as all the experts and researchers were to our cause, at the end of the day our real priority was not just to make headlines in scientific journals, but to transform people's lives. In front of us, we had the evidence that – in Balsall Common, at least – we had done that. Every single child that we had tested and identified as having as yet undiscovered potential was referred to our programme and treated. Having established this model of success, the only other question was how long would it be before other schools followed suit?

OTHER SCHOOL RESEARCH STUDIES

The success of the Balsall Common project has meant that several Education Boards have been involved in pilot projects using the programme in schools. These other studies show remarkable consistency in the results with all studies showing dramatic improvements in progress of the treated children. In summary, they demonstrate that:

- The more severe the dyslexic symptoms are, the more effective the programme has been
- Reading improvements have ranged from 200 to 400 per cent improvements compared to previous progress, the figures being higher in the more severely affected children
- Spelling has up to 200 per cent improvement compared to previous rates of progress
- There are remarkable improvements in attention ability with over 90 per cent showing improved symptoms of the attention problems commonly seen.

LARGE-SCALE STUDIES

The latest research on literally thousands of people that have gone through the programme has measured the average progress in the key indicators used to assess cognitive function using one of the most widely used dyslexia screening tests. It shows that in the year that children went through the programme the average progress in many key areas is remarkable:

- Verbal fluency – they made three times more progress than they were expected to achieve
- Phonological skills – they made more than four times the progress that they were expected to make
- Working memory – they made five times more progress than they were expected to make
- Co-ordination skills – they made six times more progress than they were expected to make

These large studies have also looked at symptoms of ADHD before and after the programme using the DSM IV classification. In both children and adults, these studies show that:

- Over 90 per cent of people have a reduction in the symptoms of both attention and hyperactivity after completing the programme
- Nearly 80 per cent show such a reduction of symptoms that previously diagnosed ADHD sufferers would no longer be classified for attention or hyperactivity problems (this is why some pronounce it a cure!)
- The effectiveness of these improvements is seen in children and adults alike.

Our other studies in the UK and Australia have shown that even a year after finishing the programme these improvements are sustained. As a result of the programme, many children on prescription medication for ADHD stopped taking their medication. Parents are often amazed and to quote one of them:

> *'I wonder if you can imagine how different it was doing the Dore Achievement Centre's exercises to doing our usual routine with David. He has great trouble with both his reading and writing; we used to get him to do a bit of extra work most days after school, and the battles and tears were just appalling. He was beginning to see himself as a failure and he was both resentful and frustrated. We were trying to help but we were not getting anywhere. Then this folder came home with his exercises. Well, right from the start he did the exercises cheerfully – hopping round the kitchen table was his favourite and throwing the beanbag up in the air. In addition, crazy as it seems, he started to get better at his reading as he progressed through the programme. That, of course, made him even keener on doing the exercises and the whole thing took off. I think David felt in control and that he was achieving for the first time.'*
>
> Marianne (mum)

So what else will we research? The (brain imaging) studies currently under way will give us further insight into what is happening in the brain. Despite my scepticism, I suspect we will soon conduct a research project that will include a control group. Until we do this, there will always be some researchers who will be holding back from embracing this breakthrough – and we really want to prove to everyone just how promising this is.

Chapter 11

ADHD – YOUNG OFFENDERS AND CRIME

Up to this point, our main focus has always been to develop ways of helping children and adults with learning difficulties. We were therefore concerned to discover just how severe life can be for people suffering from these problems. As there is significant research showing that the majority of prisoners suffer from various types of learning difficulty, in October 2002, we decided we wanted to conduct a study in a prison and were fortunate to find a prison governor who was prepared to allow us to undertake such a project.

The prison was one of those old Victorian-type prisons; a foreboding place with very high walls. It is actually quite close to the centre of the town and so casts a very dark shadow over it. The inside is even grimmer than the outside. It is a dismal and dingy place that is also very crowded. However, the prisoners are lucky that the staff have very positive attitudes, despite the conditions they have to work in.

I was introduced to the governor of the prison and I asked her

if she would allow us to carry out a research project. I explained to her that we would need a group of prisoners who were going to be there for at least 18 months, as this would help us monitor them before, during and after the programme. She invited me to give a talk to other members of the staff and I was pleased to find them very receptive and supportive of my idea. The other criterion I suggested was that I wanted to make a video of the whole process. A friend of mine, who was an ex-BBC producer, had expressed an interest in recording everything with a view to making a documentary. I thought this was a great idea, but it did present us with one important problem: we would need to find a group of prisoners who would not cause an adverse reaction if their faces were to be shown on television. Therefore, we would not be able to use prisoners who had been involved in a crime against another person, such as rape or grievous bodily harm. The governor could not see a problem with this idea and duly set up a meeting for me to address a group of prisoners to gauge their interest.

As I was driving up the motorway for this meeting, it dawned on me that this would be one of the hardest talks I had ever been asked to give. Standing up in front of an audience and telling them about our treatment was always something I looked forward to, as it gave me a chance to give people some hope. Even when dealing with a sceptical audience, I enjoyed the challenge of responding to criticism and seeing the change in people's attitudes as I explained to them how their as yet unlocked potential could be accessed. I remember feeling nervous that I might get a hostile and negative reaction from these prisoners; this feeling of unease turned out to be justified.

A group of about 50 prisoners was assembled in the prison chapel. Even before I stood up, I could see that their body

language was one of total disinterest. Apparently, they only came to hear me as it meant they got two hours off from making mail sacks. I had never before met prisoners in a prison. If I had, I expect this would have been much less of a surprise. I was probably 20 minutes into my speech before it became clear that my tactics were not working: no one was looking at me, or showing the slightest bit of interest or concern. They were simply waiting for me to finish so they could go back to whatever activity they were to go back to next; it was dreadfully hard work.

Finally, I decided to completely abandon my normal style and to try to engage with them. I had a breakthrough when I asked the question 'Is anyone good at soccer?' A lone voice in the crowd replied, 'Where the **** do you think we can play football in here, mate?' The voice belonged to a man in his late twenties. His arms were folded and he clearly had a downhearted, morose attitude. He did not even look up to speak; he just sat there with his head bowed. So I asked him if he liked soccer, to which he lethargically replied, 'Yeah – I have got OK skills, but I am not really good at it.' I then did my best to explain to him what might be happening when he was playing. I said that, while it was probable that he might have some good ball skills, these were likely to suffer when he had to make a quick decision. I told him that guys like him quite often prefer to be the striker or the goalie rather than a midfield player – this is because they find it easier to focus their minds on one single objective.

After I finished speaking, there was a brief pause before he replied, 'How the **** did you know that, mate? You're bang on!'

A disconcerted mumble went through the crowd. Suspicions were raised that I had been talking to the prison staff to get this information on him.

Despite this, I continued, 'I guess you missed a lot of school,

too, because you hated the whole process. I bet you felt like you had some good ideas inside you and sensed that you were brighter than some of the others in your class but for some reason you could never get those ideas down on paper so you always came out badly in tests and exams?'

For the first time, he actually lifted his eyes to look at me. This time he did not swear, he just looked at me with startled eyes and asked, 'How did you know that?'

Together, we talked through his whole school experience, about how he had felt he had a good brain but was caged in by his ability to get information into and out of his brain.

For each dissenting voice that rose out of the crowd, I asked that person a line of questions to get them communicating. Within the next 15 minutes, I had opened up a dialogue with a number of prisoners, who were amazed how I could explain what life was like at school for them, the social problems they had, their difficulties with reading, and so on. By the end of the talk, my shirt was soaking with sweat, but I had at least managed to just about get through to them: all bar one of that group agreed to participate in the research project – so far, so good!

GETTING STARTED

We arranged for a few of the prisoners to be filmed talking about their lives and their expectations of the programme. This was a very interesting process. It was amazing how many of them thought that our programme was likely to make them better criminals. They thought it would make them more astute, more devious and give them the cunning and guile necessary to help them avoid being caught in the future. Some of these prisoners, of course, did not want to show their face when they were filmed so it was agreed that they were to be pixellated out in the

documentary. But not everyone had such a cynical viewpoint. Many of the prisoners told us the most amazing stories. They felt that we were beginning to explain how they could be so bright underneath, yet perform so poorly academically. This, of course, had been a block for them getting any serious job.

So the whole group started their exercises and we watched them with great interest, keen to see how they would perform. We soon realised that life in prison is not easy for anyone, not least of all the wardens. The logistical challenges they face to get prisoners to do what they should do each day were interesting to witness. Several of those who had intended to start the programme did not manage to stick at it for more than a few days at a time. Yet surprisingly many of the prisoners complied with little or no fuss. Some eventually saw this as something that could really help them and others simply viewed it as temporary respite to doing laborious prison work.

PROBLEMS

Just as we thought we were making some headway, an unprecedented event happened that was to have a detrimental impact on our whole experiment. Within a few months of us starting the programme, there was a change in the classification of prisoners the authorities wished to hold at the prison. This meant that many of those in the group were moved to other jails, making it impossible for them to continue with the programme. Consequently, our group of committed prisoners was whittled down to a much smaller contingent.

As if this was not problematic enough, the prison had gone through some building changes, which resulted in the lowering of the height of the archway gate, under which we had been moving our mobile equipment. This was catastrophic and the only way we

could get round it was by carrying our heavy equipment into the prison. It was a very slow and laborious process and I was petrified something would be damaged.

All of these things were outside of the control of the governor of the prison and the staff, who were wonderfully co-operative. Nevertheless, it was a maddeningly frustrating time for all of us involved and I worried about how this untimely change in legislation was going to affect the significance of what we were trying to achieve. Nevertheless, we soldiered on, hoping we would see the sorts of changes that would make the whole ordeal worthwhile.

RESULTS

After six months, when the day finally came to access the group's progress, all of us involved were sorry that the experiment was coming to an end. But we had encountered so many unforeseen obstacles and challenges that the Balsall Common School experiment was beginning to feel like a walk in the park. However, when I finally met with the small remaining group who had gone all the way through the programme, all of these problems seemed petty and irrelevant: the change that had taken place was enormous. They were communicative and supportive of each other and keen to speak up and tell the group stories about the changes they had experienced over the months.

One Jamaican inmate, for instance, said that he had started writing songs. As he said this, there was a chorus of supportive comments from the other prisoners about the quality of the music he had been writing since he started doing the exercises. In fact, prior to going through the programme, he had not been able to compose anything. Suddenly, it was as if a fog had been lifted, and words and melodies were just flowing from him.

Another inmate spoke about the fact that, prior to being put in jail, he had never been able to pass his electrician's exams. He had asked one of his supervisors whether he was allowed to take them now that he had completed our programme and they had replied, 'What's the point? You haven't been doing any studying!' Despite this, he persisted in his request and was eventually granted his wish. He passed the exams with distinction! Clearly, our programme had not taught him anything. However, what we did do was to give him the ability to access the information that was already in his brain in a way that was far faster and more effortless than he had ever been able to do before.

One young man still in his twenties who had claimed at the beginning of the course that the programme would make him a better criminal changed his mind completely. By now, he had decided that he was going to become a personal trainer and had got a clear plan for the rest of his life. Some months later, in September 2004, when the UK centres were having their annual conference the same man gave a speech. His self-esteem had improved; he was able to read, to study, to concentrate, to get on with people around him, and so on. It was not until the end that someone asked him where he lived. During his talk, he had never mentioned that he was still in prison for a crime and when he replied that he was still in prison a huge gasp went around the room.

Amazingly, all the prisoners who complied with the programme had made substantial progress in many practical ways. They had thrilled us by their transformation and they had surprised themselves. Of course, some of them had missed so much schooling in their early life that they had never learned the basic skills necessary for reading and writing. For these inmates, the hole in the bucket had been plugged and now all that was needed

was some basic teaching so it could be filled. As a result of what was observed in the prison, some of the staff signed up to do the programme and put their children on it, too.

So what was the sum total of what we achieved? The results we had seen had given me much encouragement that our programme might one day help solve many of the problems faced by governments in the fight against crime. Anecdotally, we had seen that these simple exercises could help improve an offender's quality of life by providing them with a sense of purpose, by reducing their frustrations and giving them the ability to read, write, communicate and concentrate. These qualities are essential if a person is to have any chance of conducting a useful life that in some way contributes to society. At a human and at an economic level, we must investigate this opportunity further.

But I have learned an important lesson; when doing any further research that involves the co-operation of a government department, I will only support it financially if they do likewise.

DELINQUENCY

Not long ago, I was approached by one of the inspectors from Avon and Somerset Police Force. One of his colleagues had observed the remarkable changes that people going through our programme had experienced and wanted us to research whether our treatment might help persistent young offenders. With delinquency, or the ASBO (Anti-Social Behaviour Order) system, as it is sometimes called in the UK, being such an issue now, the pressure really is on us to see whether we can make a difference. According to a government count, anti-social behaviour happens every two seconds. The count, over a 24-hour period on 10 September 2004, found 66,107 recorded incidents of anti-social behaviour (ASB). Consequently, it has

become one of the most talked-about issues in Parliament, and the UK government has even set up a new anti-social behaviour unit at the Home Office.

We discussed this with the police authority who arranged for a substantial grant to be obtained so we could carry out the project appropriately. Thus, we were able to begin.

As it is early days, it may still be too soon to draw any conclusions. However, since my last chat with the inspector, it seems that all those complying with the programme bar one seem to have improved their behaviour and have virtually stopped committing crimes – very encouraging. Only time will tell whether we can make a real difference to the lives of these young folk: I really hope we can.

We know already that the single biggest issue that young people have is that they need someone to mentor them so that they are motivated to do an exercise programme for a year or so. Without such mentoring, few would comply. But, with so much to gain, surely there must be a way to achieve that – even at the economic level it makes sense. One day some economic advisor to the government will work out the sums.

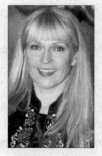

TOYAH WILLCOX?S STORY

'My life changed immediately and dramatically in November 2003 following a revolutionary treatment called the Dore Programme, which I believe has subdued my dyslexia to the point of appearing cured. I've been so bowled over by it that I now want to tell everybody about it.'

In her 30-year career, Toyah Willcox has written over 18 albums, won awards around the world, made over ten feature films and has appeared in over 30 stage plays. She managed to achieve all this despite the fact she had learning difficulties. Once again, this illustrates that, just because a person suffers from dyslexia or ADHD, it does not have any reflection whatsoever on their intelligence. Nevertheless, even with all her achievements, Toyah still felt as if she had not achieved her full potential. This is her story in her own words.

'Growing up with learning difficulties can be an extremely painful, frustrating and lonely experience for many people. When you are failing academically and struggling to express yourself in social situations, it is so easy to fall into the trap of believing you are stupid or thick. However, hopefully people will now realise that learning difficulties are caused by a neurological problem. Being dyslexic does not mean you are stupid or lazy, it literally means that your cerebellum is underperforming. This is a problem that affects many, many people. It's so easy to feel isolated and

alone when you have a learning difficulty, but the truth is that millions are in the same boat.'

Before the Dore Programme

'It may sound like a cliché, but I wish I had known what I know now when I was at school. If I was going to school today, I expect someone would have spotted that I was, in fact, dyslexic. They would have noticed my spelling and reading were abnormal, they would have noticed that I had problems with articulation. Sadly for me, though, this didn't happen. When I was growing up, learning difficulties were not widely talked about. No one ever accepted that because I had a problem reading that I could, in fact, have an amazing IQ. Instead, I was always patronised with sympathetic looks, which said, "Never mind then."

'The truth is that I did, in fact, have a very high IQ. I was one of the brightest when it came to artistic ideas and my teachers would encourage my special skills. Nevertheless, nobody picked up on the fact that something was holding me back. Even now, it's hard to express what it feels like knowing you are different, but not knowing why. I didn't want to not fit in at school; I didn't want to be a slow learner. More than anything, I wanted to be "normal". I felt very misunderstood; people probably thought I was just lazy.

'Deep down I knew I was clever but I couldn't always articulate myself very well. When I was very young, in conversations, I always struggled to convey my thoughts and went off on tangents. My communication skills were

so bad that, whenever I tried to express myself, I would often get tongue-tied and confused. At the time, David Bowie was using the "cut-up" method to write lyrics. He took sentences, chopped them up, muddled them up and put them back together again. I actually thought and spoke like that, and when I used to try to say something it would come out in a similar jumble. I greatly admired the girls with sparkling repartee, the ones everyone always listened to. In my head, I had equal ideas to them, but they just didn't come out of my mouth.

'To help me get through school I had to develop my own coping strategies. I even invented my own ways of spelling and reading. Because I couldn't rely on total spontaneity I'd rehearse a conversation, such as mentioning a newspaper heading and saying, "Isn't this story fascinating?" to pretend I'd read it. I later used these techniques to learn stock phrases for interviews and auditions.

'Spelling was a nightmare and I also found reading was incredibly difficult. In fact, I couldn't read a book because it was just a blur of lines to me. I remember feeling as if, no matter how hard I tried, I just couldn't learn things. In the end, I was left alone by the teachers because I was just so slow at reading, writing and maths.

'It was because of these problems, I'm embarrassed to admit, that I became a bully. I was disruptive and could not be controlled by the teachers. The real pity was that my father had spent a lot of money sending me to a private school and I wasn't able to make the most of the opportunity. When I wasn't causing trouble, I would be

staring blankly out of the window completely oblivious to what was going on in the classroom.

'Even as an adult these problems stayed with me. I remember filming Quadrophenia *in 1979 with Sting, and he was teaching me how to sing the backing vocals to The Police hit "Roxanne". They were simple and famous harmonies, but I couldn't visualise the music or hear the rhythm. So I ended up smashing furniture around the room and banging my fist down on tables, saying, "Sting, I will never learn it – I can't learn in the normal way!" He didn't know I was dyslexic nor did I admit it.*

'Nevertheless, I did manage to excel in other ways: I had a very successful career and worked extremely hard. In many ways, I felt that I had overcome my problems – I accepted who I was, and I led a very fulfilling life.'

On the Dore Programme

'I found out about the Dore Programme in November 2003. Having got to a point in my life where I had accepted I would have to live with dyslexia, it was quite a shock to hear that this treatment had already helped thousands overcome their learning difficulties. I knew that I had to try the programme for myself.

'I started with some basic exercises, such as spinning in a circle and then trying to sit on a big gym ball. If I had tried to spin around three years ago, I would have been sick – apparently, many dyslexics and dyspraxics suffer from travel sickness, a sign that the cerebellum isn't working as it should. I did my exercises religiously for

three months, twice a day. The effects were immediate. My life improved within a week of starting the exercises. It was as if suddenly the dam wall started to come down. All of those thoughts and ideas that had once been a jumbled mess inside of my head were starting to connect and take shape. Some people I have spoken to, who have also been through the programme, say that they have noticed exactly the same thing: it's as if a fog has been lifted from your eyes and suddenly you have been given the power to articulate yourself far more clearly than ever before.

'I expect many people who do not suffer from learning difficulties will find it hard to appreciate just how liberating it feels to suddenly be able to communicate in the way you have always wanted to, without having to worry about getting confused or frustrated. All I can say is that it is like being given a second chance. So many people get to the point where they believe they know themselves and know their own limits. Then they do the Dore Programme and suddenly everything is turned on its head. All those things that were always a struggle suddenly become much easier; all of those barriers that prevent you from achieving your full potential disappear.

'Since the exercises began to take effect, I have hardly stopped writing. This is pretty incredible considering writing was once the bane of my life. I have also noticed that my spelling has improved dramatically. Now I feel my life is speeding up. In the past I'd have days of being completely frozen in a creative mental block and unable to do anything. My dyslexia had a terrible effect on my songwriting. If I had

creative moments, they lasted only an hour. Now the prison door is unlocked and I feel I can work whenever I want to. Even though I still have blocks on some names and certain words I can't understand or spell, I no longer get cross. In the past, the majority of my energy went on being frustrated; now I have learned that this is a wasted emotion.

'Crucially, my social skills have improved beyond belief. I used to be lonely socially and felt everyone hated me. But, within three weeks of starting the treatment, I became confident and now feel able to go up and talk to anyone. My verbal memory recall has been transformed and I can hold conversations without going off at tangents.

'My husband, guitarist Robert Fripp, cannot believe the transformation. I used to have black days filled with the frustration of not being able to read or write. At the time, I had no idea about the concept of working memory and I didn't realise that these feelings were brought on because my cerebellum wasn't doing its "librarian" job properly. Whenever I tried to write, I would have to concentrate extremely hard. If I was distracted, I would often lose my trail of thought, which could be extremely annoying and frustrating. Doing the Dore Programme corrected the problem with my cerebellum, freeing up my working memory to do its job. In essence, that means that when I am writing I can now happily turn my attention to something else without feeling overloaded or weighed down.

'In the same way, before I did the programme, if I had a negative thought in my head, I didn't have enough available working memory space left to bring in

compensatory thoughts to rationalise my feelings. Now I do. Not only has this dramatically improved my life, but I expect it has improved Robert's, too.

'The Dore Programme is not a quick fix because it takes dedication for a while. However, the course made me instantly happy. Now I've got the stepping stones to a better life. The system is also being used by many sportsmen: it is thought to be particularly helpful for sports involving hand–eye co-ordination, such as football, rugby and cricket, as it can dramatically improve players' awareness of the ball, as well as their awareness of other players on the pitch.

'Wynford plans eventually to help big business executives improve their memory and motivational skills, and is even researching balance and memory problems in old people, including reducing the effects of Alzheimer's disease. For me, it has opened a prison door I thought was locked forever. There are many ways the Dore Programme has helped me:

I'd always fly off the handle because I couldn't communicate my ideas well enough. That's gone now – my vocabulary is broadening every day.

I used to read a book once a year; now I now read a book a week. I'm getting through all the bestsellers, which I find staggering.

I now manage my own finances and spend four hours a day just on managing my investments. Several years ago, I would not have even tried to read numbers.'

Part of this account of Toyah's story first appeared in the Daily Mail *on 27 December 2005.*

Chapter 12

HOW HAS THE LEARNING DIFFICULTIES WORLD REACTED?

Back in the early days, it seemed likely to us that anybody who was anybody working in the field of learning difficulties would become as excited about our breakthrough as we were. Of course, from the beginning, many became quickly very excited, and today it is in rapidly increasing numbers. However, we looked forward to the day when government organisations and institutions around the world would embrace this science so that we could rapidly develop it further and make it widely available to everyone. Sadly, this has not yet happened in the way that we hoped and, from the moment we set up our first centre, we faced a huge barrage of criticism and unsupportive attitudes from many key players.

What many people do not seem to realise is that we are not trying to keep this breakthrough to ourselves to develop a commercial empire. The problem is far too large for only one small organisation to be pushing such an important project forward. Providing other organisations wishing to work with us are

genuine in their intent and not simply out to exploit the programme commercially, we will be happy to work with them.

NEGATIVE REACTION TO THE TREVOR MCDONALD PROGRAMME

Immediately after the television documentary went on air, I braced myself for an assault. Although I expected this to come from a few different quarters, strangely the only critics seemed to be from within the learning difficulties industry itself. Not only were they not excited about what we had done, but they had venom in their attack on us. I remember thinking back to Dr Levinson's words about the keen competitiveness of researchers and, for the first time, I could see what he meant. For years, the whole learning difficulties industry had been becoming more and more fragmented. There are a whole host of independent small institutions and clinics that have been set up through the years, all championing their own theories and ideas. As a result, the situation was one of immense competitiveness and rivalry between hundreds of different research facilities, offering nutritional programmes, drug-related treatments, reading programmes, behavioural therapy, optical solutions and so on. Each one had spent huge amounts of initiative, effort, time and money. Therefore, when we arrived on the scene, it was crowded with competing theories whose proponents were hungry for success.

One of the criticisms thrown at us was that the Trevor McDonald show had said we were a 'revolutionary breakthrough in the treatment of dyslexia'. The fact was that we were not the very first exercise programme that had come along purporting to help those with learning difficulties. However, one of the problems with most of the existing programmes was that they were based on the assumption that one size fits all and did not

take into account that every person has a different brain and therefore needs different exercises. In addition, of course, another benefit of our programme had come from the recent breakthrough in the understanding of what is happening in the brain, particularly the cerebellum. So what we were doing had only become possible in the last few years and these other exercise-based programmes had been around for a lot longer than that and were based on earlier theories. The reason we were different was that we were able to treat people according to their individual needs, needs we had been able to measure in the neurological tests. With the huge amount of wiring that takes place in the brain, it is clear that one single generic exercise is unlikely to work equally well for everyone. In the same way that people exercise differently in the gym because they are different sizes and shapes and have different goals, you cannot put the brain through a single generic workout and expect to maximise that person's full potential.

It is a sad fact that in an area like learning difficulties, where there is such a strong and desperate need, individuals and organisations are narrow-mindedly pushing their own solutions. There are insufficient resources available to tackle the problem as it is. The last thing we need is for this group of wonderful people to be fighting within itself, increasing the confusion and despair in those that need help. The hostile response shocked and appalled me. I thought they would have been thrilled at the results we were getting; I even hoped that they would see what we were doing and want to work with us. As we were about to discover repeatedly, getting this co-operation was not going to be easy.

Another area from which we received criticism was some educationalists, who for years had been promoting the use of

phonological teaching methods. These techniques had certainly improved the reading ability of some children; however, the results were hardly dramatic. In fact, scientific studies had indicated that the results were often quite poor. Typically those studies would show improvements in reading ability of a few per cent a year. We were often seeing improvements of 500 per cent in comprehension progress and 300 per cent reading progress in a year, yet we were not seeing an increase in their teaching support at all.

Once again, I was dismayed by the response, having expected the education authorities to be ecstatic that we were saying learning difficulties were rarely the fault of poor teaching. I strived to make the point that, in my experience, teachers work very, very hard. Typically, they are highly successful in getting 85 per cent of their class to learn to read and write. However, the other 15 per cent clearly have problems outside their control. Learning difficulties are usually the result of neurological and physiological problems and rarely caused by poor teaching. Despite this, educationalists responded to the programme by saying things like 'there can be no substitute for good teaching'. Effectively, this argument points the finger of blame towards the teachers – if a student is not making progress, it must be their fault. How unfair and unscientific this criticism is!

Our argument has always been that, if you correct the root problem in the brain, the same teaching will produce much better results. When you expose children to our programme, not only do they typically catch up with their peers, but also they often make more progress than those children who never had learning difficulties. This is exactly what our first research project proved.

Another criticism was that our programme is too expensive. Interestingly, this was typically from those wedded to other

theories and rarely from the families of sufferers. For me, this is obviously a very sensitive subject because the last thing I wanted was for the programme to be available only to the rich and famous, and, indeed, it is not. Yet I have always responded to these comments by asking people to seriously consider whether they truly believe it is expensive. Compare it to the price of braces for teeth, breast implants, a family holiday or upgrading your car. Surely, it is a price worth paying in the attempt to transform the life of your child so that they are able to enjoy school, to develop social skills, to develop good sporting skills, to have good prospects in life?

Strangely, the people saying we were expensive were promoting programmes that cost as much as ours, the cost to participants in many of the alternative programmes was ongoing. In real terms, many folk using these other treatments have paid several times the cost of our programme and have not seen a fraction of the results. Our programme is usually completed in 12–18 months and no further treatment is needed.

Others criticised me because they said I was a businessman looking to make a profit. Had they taken the trouble to have a look at our accounts, they would have seen that not only have I not taken a salary since the project began, but also I have happily contributed millions of pounds, year after year after year, because I want to solve this problem. To this day, I have continued to do so because there is so much costly research and development to be done.

Of course, the effect these comments had was horrific. How many people were put off contacting us may never be known, but we suspect many were consequently denied a great opportunity to transform their lives. As we know that 89 per cent of those suffering from depression have some symptoms of learning

difficulties, if we had simply said that people like Susie needed to learn to live with their difficulties, we believe passionately that not only would Susie and others like her not have been helped, but also they would be condemned to a life of misery and frustration.

THE NATURE OF PARADIGM SHIFTS

To understand why the reception to new ideas and new discoveries is often so negative, Professor David Reynolds explained to me the concept of the 'paradigm shift' and the typical reaction from both the public and those with vested interests. I am told a paradigm shift takes place when the established viewpoint of most people is changed, or altered in some way. The most crude example of this would be when Columbus discovered the world was round, a revelation that literally turned a fundamental belief on its head. Suddenly, whole societies had to re-evaluate their belief systems; nothing was ever quite the same again. So when I talk about what has now been labelled as the 'Dore Programme' in terms of a paradigm shift, it is because I believe that this breakthrough has the power to overturn most of the established ideas about learning difficulties that have gone before us.

It almost seems as if, every time there is a new discovery, the real gatekeepers to change are the scientists and researchers who exhibit a negative automatic reflex response. The problem is that paradigm shifts usually take a long while to benefit all that need it because there is always resistance to change. Amazingly, some still belong to The Flat Earth Society. I often cite the example that when ophthalmic experts first came up with the idea of eyeglasses they were laughed out of court; I wonder when history will stop repeating itself. For centuries, people have

occasionally come up with effective new treatments that for decades, and in some cases centuries, have failed to achieve recognition. As a result, generations have continued to suffer needlessly until they finally become accepted.

What happened to us was no different to what happened to the methods developed for tackling stomach ulcers many years ago by two Australian doctors, Robin Warren and Barry Marshall, who would not accept that a cure was impossible. Despite their efforts, for a long time they were shouting in the wind because the medical profession believed their theories were unsubstantial. It took ten years before their work got any serious support from medical researchers and it was 20 years before their treatment really started to be available to the general population. How many suffered because of the slow-moving machinery of change? No doubt, it was millions of people.

To me, it seems obvious that there needs to be a more scientific way of evaluating cures that have the potential to cause a paradigm shift. It scares me to think that it might be a decade or more before our treatment becomes available everywhere.

Of course, people's attitudes towards us were coloured by the fact that over the years there had been so many false dawns in the industry. Many theories, concepts and ideas had been paraded as potential panaceas for learning difficulties, but, for the majority of those who tried them, all had led to disappointment. Over the last few years, some people have been talking about them with great excitement because a few have seen some improvements in their reading. Nevertheless, the majority we have come across that have tried them seem to have been largely disappointed.

The path to acceptance was not an easy one and, around the time of the Balsall Common School project, we were becoming embroiled in all sorts of practical challenges. To drive our

substantial research programme, we needed to persuade enough people to come through the programme. Despite all the speeches I made and all the people I spoke to, only a few professionals from the learning difficulties world seemed to believe what I was telling them. The general consensus seemed to be that, at best, ours was a radical and expensive treatment that had no guarantee of success; it seemed they just did not want to face what was really being achieved.

Even Trevor Davies, the headmaster of Balsall Common, was puzzled by the fact that such stunning results had been achieved at his school and yet I had been relatively ineffective at getting the message across. He decided to do all he could to help by speaking to various headmasters around the country. Yet even he struggled to create in others the immediate mindset change that he knew the programme's results deserved.

Despite all these challenges, I never lose determination or focus. All around us, we were surrounded by examples and anecdotes of the dramatic effects our programme was having on people's lives. While it was deeply frustrating to know that we were sitting on a breakthrough few seemed to be interested in, we were constantly reminded by our patients of the importance of what we were doing. This instilled in us a great sense of drive and purpose, and gave us the oxygen we needed to keep going.

THE DANGER OF USING THE 'C' WORD

It was not long before the phrase 'miracle cure' started to be used in the media. This worn-out description seems to appear almost every time an alternative cure comes on to the market. These days there are more 'miracle cures' than 'conditions'. Indeed, every other day the papers appear full of 'breakthrough' medical advancements in skincare technology or diet regimes. It is not

surprising that the word 'cure' breeds cynicism in the minds of the public and the Establishment alike.

The simple fact is the programme is no more a 'miracle cure' than a painkiller is. In fact, it is probably far less miraculous. Having said this, whether you want to label the programme a 'breakthrough' or 'miracle' cure, certainly it was progress and everyone involved knew it was something extremely special and out of the ordinary. While many others were using these words to describe our results, we chose not to. Despite this, some so-called experts remained unimpressed. Instead, we were criticised because others were saying this of us! Some professionals will always associate 'miracle cure' with organisations that are, in some way or another, shady. Often, I have spoken quite sarcastically about how some medical researchers seem to take great pride in exclaiming at the top of their voices that 'there is no such thing as a cure for learning difficulties!' If that is the case, why is it that they are given money for research funding? The fact is that, if they are not actually looking for a cure, it is extremely unlikely they will ever find one.

We have always been looking for something that will, in effect, be a cure and have never made any secret of this, even though we have been slow to consider using the word. The reason why some of the professors writing up our research reports now use the word 'cure' is clear. Not only have they seen the programme help a large proportion of those people that complete it overcome their leaning difficulties, but also, a year or so afterwards, they have witnessed them continuing to make the same remarkable progress. This is the complete opposite of other methods, where typically people show signs of regression after finishing a course.

The debate is still on. Should we use the word 'cure'? On the

other hand, ought we to pander to certain elements of the learning difficulties community and avoid using it? Of course, I would prefer to be completely straightforward and it is the most apt description, but I am conscious this might offend some people. In the end, we must persuade everyone of our success so we might have to temper our language to be more modest for a while. Our current view is that, if other people want to use the word 'cure', we are happy for them to do so. But we believe that the symptoms we are dealing with are not the result of a disease but incomplete development. So, if it isn't a disease, it can't be cured. But, if you can complete the development, let others reach their own conclusion as to which words should be used to describe the process. I suspect the debate will last at least a couple of decades. As long as those that need help don't have to wait too long.

SCIENTIFIC REACTION TO OUR RESEARCH PROJECT

Apparently, it is quite usual for breakthrough research to be lambasted by other scientists. Every time a project is completed or results are published, there is always someone waiting to criticise, judge and undermine. While I am sure many have quite sincere motives, the intentions of others might be called into question. Sadly, it is often the case that many are just interested in making a name for themselves rather than supporting scientific and medical progress. While the importance of scrutiny and the expression of legitimate arguments should always be upheld, all too often, certain parties are more interested in adding to their own reputations. For me, this is really poor form when it comes to derailing genuine progress.

The Balsall Common research project was a first for me. I had never done anything remotely like that before, but I was convinced that the only way the politicians would listen was if I

could show them hard, solid evidence. I assumed our findings would impress scientists and academics more than they would anyone else – I cannot believe how mistaken I was! Before our research could be published, it had to go through a process called 'peer review'. This is where a number of professors examine the findings of a report and give their verdict. The response was very interesting indeed. While there were obviously many very supportive and positive messages, there were lots of adverse comments as well.

My good friend from Warwick University, Professor Don Jenkins, gave me great comfort. For almost 20 years, I had enjoyed working with him while pioneering breakthrough research in fire-protection coatings. Professor Jenkins had written many, many research papers and warned me that criticism was to be expected for any paradigm shift. He told me I should not be worried at all and he sent me many different examples of similar cases where breakthroughs had been treated with utter contempt. Through these cases, I could see that suspicion of the new and bold often manifested itself in opposition to the point of being total warfare.

There was also the example of Professor Jeremy Schmahmann, the distinguished Researcher of Neuropsychology at Harvard Medical School. I believe it took him ten years to have his research on the cerebellum peer reviewed and published. Consequently, for a decade, researchers did not have access to this insightful information, and progress in our understanding of how the brain worked was delayed. After many more years' study, Schmahmann's work, *Fiber Pathways of the Brain*, was eventually published and its importance is realised. Indeed, he is now the noteworthy author of the first complete book on the anatomy of the brain to be published for more than 100 years.

In essence, I am rather cynical about the peer-review process when there is a paradigm shift involved. I strongly suspect it has hampered many a breakthrough for many years. It seems an awful lot easier to get minor variations on already established views through the system, whereas something new takes a lot of guts, time and persistence.

My main concern was that with such a mixed scientific reaction we would have trouble getting our message across. Nevertheless, over the next few years, we carried out more and more research projects and we will continue to do so.

THE PROGRAMME AND THE BRITISH GOVERNMENT

We always assume governments are armed with all the information they need to make perfect decisions all the time. Of course, as we saw in the run-up to the war with Iraq, this is not always the case. Government departments rely upon advisers to give them the latest information so that they can make good decisions. One of the problems with learning difficulties is that for decades it has been regarded as an educational problem, hence this is where the focus has been and it is, to a major extent, educationalists who seem to have had a major influence in the decision-making process. What we now know is that the root cause of the problem is a physiological one and must be corrected first by using physiological means before any educational programmes will have their full effect. While I have been frustrated in the past by the lack of government interest in what we are doing, I am hopeful that in ten years' time government advisory committees will have a better mix of educationalists, psychologists, neurologists and physiologists. This could make a world of difference.

I have also been frustrated that there is no government in the

world that I know of that, as a standard practice, screens every child early in their school life to find out if they have learning difficulties. I expect this is because, up until now, there has been very little governments felt they could do about the problem. Hence, why would they want to bring attention to it?

For years, the government had thrown millions into improving teaching methods to help students with learning difficulties and particularly with poor reading skills. One of the methods they backed involved using phonics to help children with their reading and writing. Despite years of research and investment, there was very little evidence to suggest it was working really well. On the other hand, while most phonological methods may show an improvement of a few per cent in the rate of progress in reading, in our programme we were seeing a 300 per cent increase in the progress of reading age and a 500 per cent increase for comprehension.

Our first meeting with the Department of Education was actually a very pleasant one. It had followed several failed attempts to set up a meeting, but finally in 2003 they agreed to sit down with us and talk. They were very professional and supportive; however, I got the distinct impression that nothing much was going to happen quickly as a consequence. The government machine is a very big one and the cogs work very slowly indeed. With most of the advisers on this subject being educationalists, the chances of them advocating a physiological intervention into the system were very slim. We were told to go off and get some more research, which is precisely what we did.

We were not, of course, told precisely what research studies to do. Had they done that, it would have meant that, after we had carried out the research and brought it back to them, they would not have been able to tell us it was insufficient. This is typical of discussions with high-ranking government officials; when we

present our reports, which show stunning results, we anticipate it will be the start of an exciting new era. What we find is that people who tell us to go off and get lots more data will actually change their story. When we return, they do not want to believe what we are showing them.

Having such wonderful results but failing to get the ear of government is very frustrating. We had done everything researchers had suggested: I had wonderful engineers creating software to capture the data from all our centres around the world and analyse it. I had the backing of professors and other researchers who had carried out independent research projects and I had commissioned several other reports as well. You would be hard pressed to find any other organisation in the world with more information than we had.

Some time later, I arranged for a professional firm of lobbyists to produce literature that they thought would be effective in communicating with government officials and Members of Parliament. So we produced a comprehensive, professional brochure written in a language that would mean something to MPs. It told them about the issues, it gave them the science behind what we were doing and it explained the implications for the economy. To try to get their ear, we went through absolutely everything we could think of. We sent the brochure to every MP, every member of the House of Lords and every civil servant. Despite all this, we barely produced a ruffle. Out of the many hundreds of brochures we sent out, we only had two responses. Sadly, it seemed a waste of time but I still remain confident that, when the government realises the implications of the breakthrough on so many difficult parts of society, then they will eventually beat a path to our door, but how many will have to suffer meanwhile.

A MEETING WITH GORDON BROWN

Over the years, I had got to know Toronto's famous tenor John McDermott, who had become a friend. John was fascinated with our programme and he passionately wanted us to open a centre in his home city (a project that we are now working on). Not only was he a good friend, but also he was determined to make sure many of his own very influential friends got to hear about our work. When he was invited to Chancellor Gordon Brown's house for a party, he immediately thought of me and arranged for me to be invited as a guest, too.

As is the case with someone as large as life as John, he stayed to the small hours and so we were there until most of the guests had left. I am so glad I did because it gave me the opportunity to see the real Gordon Brown. As more and more people filtered out of his house, I was able to chat with him briefly in the homely and unpretentious surroundings of his own kitchen. At that time, the Chancellor had just had his first child and was experiencing the joys of fatherhood. Had his child been a little older, I think he may well have found it much easier to take in and share the concerns I was trying to communicate to him about the traumas of having a child struggling with school. He offered me the chance to speak to one of his advisers, who he said was more knowledgeable about the subject than he was – and we are still waiting to see if any initiatives will come from that.

Government is a very big machine; it has its own agenda. Understandably, it has to be very cautious. The last thing they would want is to get involved with something that has great risk attached to it, or is otherwise ill founded. It is far easier to procrastinate and delay before looking in detail at any new breakthrough until its merits have been thoroughly evaluated over a long period of time. This may explain their reticence to get

involved with us right now. I have now stopped expecting politicians to get excited about what we are doing. The strategy we now have to take is to get the programme to as many parents and teachers as possible. Gradually, this tide will build up and reach the point where the government will be forced to act – I just hope another generation is not wasted while we wait.

My local MP, John Maples in Stratford upon Avon, was very helpful indeed. He got the point and the potential impact straight away and wrote a letter to the Minister of Health. I thought his letter was excellently written and demanded attention. However, I received the most pitiful response, suggesting that I contact the Autistic Society. Although clearly the Autistic Society carries out great work, it only covers one small aspect of the whole spectrum of learning difficulties. Not only this, but they do not have the resources to analyse what we are doing and comment on it. It puzzles me that seemingly bright people in positions of power fail to grasp such important concepts. Of course, the government has to spend its time tackling thousands of issues, but why is it that, when it comes to this particular issue, they constantly choose to sweep it under the carpet and delegate it out to external agencies?

One day, the government will realise the enormous impact that we will have on the economy. They may not appreciate the impact at the human level, but, when they realise that 85 per cent of prisoners have learning difficulties and that a large proportion of the long-term unemployed and drug addicts has learning difficulties, they will understand that the cost of this issue to the economy is enormous. One day, we will transform this problem and the sooner they realise it, the better for them and for those who suffer.

THE NEED FOR BENCHMARKING

One of the consequences of there being so much argument and disagreement amongst the learning difficulty experts themselves was that, when the government was looking for ways to help people with learning difficulties, no clear message was getting through. With so many conflicting theories and ideas flying about it, it is not really surprising that the government did not take much of an interest in our discovery. Not only were different theories abundant, but the very definitions of dyslexia, dyspraxia, Asperger's Syndrome and ADHD are by no means clear-cut either.

As I discussed earlier, there is so much overlap between these conditions that it is sometimes near impossible to make distinctions. Many organisations seemed to have their own set of definitions for what learning difficulties actually were, making comprehension of the subject almost impossible.

Substantial testing of drug-based treatments and reading programmes has taken place for sufferers of ADHD and dyslexia. These, however, are only intended to address just some of the large number of symptoms that these problems bring with them. To cover all of the aspects that sufferers would like to see improve, a comprehensive benchmarking system needs to be developed. With the advent of what we are achieving with such a wide range of symptoms we must and, therefore, we will, need to become a powerful lobby group, or the full impact of what we are achieving will never be measured, let alone understood.

It soon occurred to me that the only way we were going to make ourselves stand out was if we could benchmark the programme against other methods used to tackle it. Unfortunately, there was no such protocol in place that would allow us to do so. This is, of course, a real problem for the millions of teachers and parents who, when faced with the responsibility

of looking after a child with learning difficulties, do not know where to turn. They are posed with a huge variety of options, but have no way of knowing which one is going to work best for them. Clearly, what is needed is a defined quality standard to evaluate and report on whether a treatment programme is safe, effective and suitable. You would not drive a car unless you knew it had been quality controlled during manufacture – you want to know that the brakes work, the steering works, the locks work, and so on. Quality control is a standard practice and a way of life for all products and services these days – why not for education, too?

As soon as we realised this, we started to work on what we could do to try to make it happen. I worked with Professor Rod Nicolson trying to get all the key movers and shakers from the dyslexic world together. I thought that through our discussions we would be able to build some bridges and find ways that all our respective theories and ideas could complement one another. On several occasions, I approached those offering educational-type programmes to see whether they would do a joint research project with us. I offered to fund it and I tried to persuade them by assuring them that their methods would be shown to be far more effective when combined with our physiological treatment. You might not be surprised to read that my suggestions fell on deaf ears and I never had any takers.

The truth of the situation is that most are frightened of benchmarking. They realise the risk they take that the results from testing their theories or programmes may not be that impressive. If you do not repair the hole in the bucket before you fill it, it is a pretty thankless task. Despite this, from day one, our organisation has taken a very serious approach to research and data analysis so that people can gain a clear understanding of what we are doing and achieving. Indeed, I believe we have

collected far more research data and testing than probably any other organisation in this field. We now have a huge database with the information that allows us to see a clear and consistent picture of what we are doing. This means that, when someone comes to us, we can tell him or them what they can realistically expect, which is a great comfort to them.

I sincerely hope it won't be long before we can insist on benchmarking for all learning difficulties programmes so that we can take away much of the emotion and mystique that surrounds the subject. This will allow people to make informed decisions about what is best for them. We only live our life once; children only have one opportunity at school. We need to make sure they are given absolutely the best opportunities available to suit their needs at the earliest possible age.

THE BRITISH DYSLEXIA ASSOCIATION AND THE FUTURE

What frustrated me most about the government's reaction was that I had so much evidence and yet they would not believe the programme was even worth looking at. In my moments of deepest frustration, I wished I could just bypass the whole system and make it available in all schools and institutions myself. It was around this time that I caught my first glimpse of light at the end of the tunnel.

The British Dyslexia Association (BDA) is an umbrella organisation in the UK that sees its role as helping to raise general awareness about dyslexia and to encourage society to be more 'dyslexia friendly'. For someone concerned about the problem, they are often the first point of contact. On their website, they summarise their position as follows:

The BDA's role has been raising awareness of the evidence and effects of dyslexia. We now also aim to develop and encourage services that meet the needs of dyslexic people. In this way, we will shape services to meet need.

As the umbrella organisation, we want dyslexic people to view the BDA as the organisation that best represents them. So the work of the BDA must reflect the values that dyslexic people hold dear.

We will listen to, and act upon, the needs of dyslexic people. We will foster a feeling of togetherness for all of our membership and respect for dyslexic people, volunteers and staff.

When you consider that in the UK learning difficulties affect at least one in six of the population, you would expect the BDA head office to be large and bristling with lots of research funds and resources to tackle this problem. Yet, even to this day, it is the exact opposite. It is a poorly funded and under-resourced institute that has somehow managed to get by with virtually no financial support from the government. It does, however, happen to have a wonderful army of staff who are prepared to put in the hours to help the organisation survive. Some of these workers are unpaid volunteers who are unfazed by the everyday frustrations that go hand in hand with the work they do. Over the years, they have worked relentlessly hard to raise awareness of the problem dyslexia entails and the enormity of it.

It would be fair to say, though, that our relationship with the BDA has not always been a smooth one. When I went to meet the then chief executive, Steve Alexander, about benchmarking in 2002, we could not agree the best solution, even though we both

felt passionately about the issue. When the BDA's subsequent chief executive, Professor Susan Tresman, took over the reins of power in 2005, things began to happen. Professor Tresman had a fresh understanding of the problems she faced and a vision of where things ought to be going. She looked at the research and the results we were getting; she also looked into criticism that we were just another commercial venture trying to make a quick buck and, before long, she started to discuss how the BDA and Dore could work together more closely.

Interestingly, Professor Tresman told me that, in her view, it is often not research studies that make a government sit up and take notice, but actually the case studies, the anecdotal evidence. She predicts that one day someone senior in government will witness what happens to a child when put through our programme and that is more likely to be the catalyst for change and action than any number of scientific studies. As she is a researcher herself, I strongly suspect she may be right. Until that day comes, we will keep trying, we will keep sending the government our latest research, and one day the truth will dawn on them.

At the time of writing, the BDA has sadly seen Professor Tresman leave her post and another chief executive is in the process of being appointed. Hopefully, the new vision will be continued, the association will start to receive the funding they need and they will broaden their role to embrace the breakthrough, and the implications it may have on the lives of the dyslexic sufferers they want to help.

Chapter 13

THE PRACTICAL RESULTS OF GOING THROUGH THE PROGRAMME

Most people find it incredible that such seemingly simple exercises could make such a difference – in fact, many times, an enormous difference – and it doesn't seem to matter at what age someone goes through the programme. Many (sometimes all) of the symptoms improve regardless of age! The fact is that for most people this programme works wonderfully and I have often met parents who comment that their children had inherited their symptoms, but, having gone through the programme, the children have lost the symptoms that the parents themselves sadly still have! So, without such a programme these symptoms rarely go away of their own accord. As someone gets older, they usually do not just grow out of it.

In the first few weeks, the exercises start working on a subtle level. They are actively building, and co-ordinating, pathways in the brain yet you will not be aware it is happening until you see the results. When learning to ride a bike, we are not aware of what happens in our brains. However, the process of moving our body

so that we stay upright (and do not fall off) gradually becomes automatic so that, after we master the skill, we can ride without thinking about balancing at all. What the exercise programme does is to replicate many of the steps of development in the brain that for some reason was not completed during the early months of life.

HOW QUICKLY DO CHANGES OCCUR?

This depends on lots of factors. If the programme is not complied with regularly, it will take far longer to complete. Here, we must sympathise: many families already have a hectic life before squeezing in an exercise programme as well, even if it is only a few minutes, into the beginning and end of each day. But clearly the programme works more quickly when done consistently, so this compliance is important. Of course, another factor is the degree of rewiring or development that is needed. Some experience a lot of progress in the first few weeks and then steady progress for the rest of the programme, whereas, for others, nothing seems to happen for ages and then, whoosh, they are off! But, as long as the desired progress happens in the end, everyone is pleased.

DO THE EFFECTS LAST?

Perhaps you are wondering about the long-term effects of this programme. After all, in the past we have seen the effects of many so-called 'breakthrough' treatments wear off in the long term. We are of course constantly studying what happens in the years after this programme has finished. Well, so far studies show that not only are the benefits retained (we presume and hope forever), but also research shows that they continue to make progress at a faster rate than others of their age who never had a learning

issue. Could this be a further clue as to how much intelligence is often hidden behind the mask?

To illustrate this point further, it is worth considering the following example. Think back to the first time you tried to ride a bike. When you sat on the saddle, the only thought running through your mind was probably something like 'I mustn't fall off!' You were not thinking about what you were doing, how you should be sitting – all you cared about was making it a few metres down your street without breaking your leg. While you were busy trying to stay upright, your brain was working to learn all it could about the skills of balance and co-ordination necessary for you to ride. It was taking that information and storing it so that gradually these skills became effortless and automatic, enabling you to ride from A to B without falling off. If you then left your bike in the shed for ten years and tried to ride it again, would you be able to? Of course! As soon as you got on it and pedalled, you would be away. The point is that you do not have to relearn something hardwired into the brain. This process of wiring is exactly what we help people to do. Once a skill has been developed and indexed properly, it is normally there for life.

FIRST CHANGES

Most people say the first differences they start to notice in themselves are that they feel less tired at the end of the day. Why is this? Because now there are more of those everyday things happening automatically with less mental effort. They also feel more enthusiastic and better about themselves (their self-esteem is higher). Often this is even before they notice any improvement in their performance and is probably caused by improved automaticity in the process of listening and speaking so they can communicate and socialise with much less effort.

CHANGES IN CHILDREN

Whether or not they know that a child is actually doing this programme, teachers sometimes detect change early on, and report back excitedly to parents. They frequently notice that a child:

- Begins to find reading easier to cope with
- Is more confident with writing and produces more written work with less heartache
- Starts to participate more in class – answering questions and expressing their ideas with more confidence
- Works better with classmates and socialises more freely
- Pays attention for longer periods and responds with enthusiasm even at the end of the day when previously they would be too tired and grouchy to work
- Is less disruptive, stays seated during class and does not call out inappropriate comments
- Joins in team games with more enthusiasm and performs better at sports involving hand-to-eye or foot-to-eye co-ordination and balance.

'Ed was a nine-year-old nightmare! He clearly struggled with the work but, instead of concentrating, he used to spend his time bugging the other kids. I could tell he was bright, but his grades were poor and his reading and writing were way behind his peer group. His parents told me they were starting him on an exercise programme but, to be honest, I did not pay much attention. I couldn't see that it would make any difference. Well, I was so happy to be proved wrong. The changes were gradual at first. I noticed I did not have to tell him off so often; he was

making better eye contact and he started progressing through the reading programme faster. His handwriting became regular and kept to the lines. One day, he showed me a story he had written at home. I was amazed: this was a child who previously took an hour to complete a paragraph of class work. Sure, it was not perfect, but his enthusiasm shone through. I put it on the wall. He was so proud he brought his parents in to show them!'
Joanne Mills, teacher

Parents are with their children every day and may not always notice gradual improvements until something happens to make them sit up and take notice. So it is with the changes that take place during the development of the cerebellum. They may not notice the academic improvement, for example, until the teacher makes them aware of it – perhaps after a test or a piece of work has been marked. In most cases, however, they do tell us that their child's mood improves fairly quickly and the atmosphere in the whole house gets better as a result. Many parents find their children are:

- Sleeping better
- More co-operative in the home
- Kinder to their brothers and sisters
- More prepared to take responsibility
- Better organised and tidier
- Better at time-keeping
- Happier and more contented
- Less volatile and moody
- Getting on with their homework and music practice with less conflict

- Eating better
- Making friends more easily
- Playing more sports
- Increasing in confidence

'I used to take my son out at weekends to practise throwing and catching a ball – well, me throwing and him missing. It was pretty demoralising and I was starting to wonder if it was doing him more harm than good. Then one day, about three weeks into the programme, he caught the ball! I just stopped running; I was so amazed. I said, "Mike, you did it! You actually caught it!" He looked at me with this big grin on his face. That was the turning point. Since then it's just got better every day.'

Gerald, paediatrician

'Before, I used to dread him coming in – he was so tired and angry. When he comes home from school now, he's bursting with energy and cannot wait to tell me his news. He's taken up distance running after school and can now do two miles in 15 minutes. For a boy who used to be terrified of trying anything new, it is a fantastic achievement!'

Marcia, mum

The children themselves have a different insight. For the first time, some of them are feeling more confident about themselves. As well as the changes they feel in themselves, they notice that people around them respond to them in a different way. They say that:

- They are making new friends
- They feel like starting new sports and hobbies

- They are finding their schoolwork easier and are keen to show how well they can do
- They are getting picked for sports teams

CHANGES IN ADULTS

Often, adults who go on a programme are already established in chosen careers that do not involve much reading and writing, so they will only become aware of improvements in their reading ability if they change their established habits and deliberately try to read and write. Moreover, frequently they then surprise themselves. Recently, I received a call from a client, Simon, who had just completed the programme. The therapist had told him he was ready to try to read. He had asked his wife's advice on what he should read and she told him that everyone was reading *The Da Vinci Code* but that he should perhaps try something simpler at first. When he spoke to me, he told me with excitement that he had just read Dan Brown's bestseller from cover to cover. There were tears in my eyes. He then went on to describe the pain he had endured when his children had been growing up and he had been unable to read to them. Prior to going on the programme, he would walk past bookshops and not even dare to turn his eyes to look in. The day before he spoke to me, he had taken the bold step of going in to Waterstone's just to experience the thrill of walking along the aisles of books and take in some of the titles that, previously, would have been beyond him, but were now completely within his grasp.

The differences adults notice vary greatly, though their partners and colleagues are often the first to report changes in the way they behave or approach their work. Adults often find that they:

- Are more relaxed
- Remember people's names better

- Keep better track of their belongings, such as keys, mobile phones and bills
- Find meetings easier to handle
- Prioritise tasks better
- Get praised at work for their performance
- Do not get so irritable at home
- Have more energy
- Read, write and fill in forms more easily
- Write and structure reports far more effortlessly

'I used to make all kinds of excuses to avoid having to write in front of my clients. I'd just make a couple of notes for each job, remember as much as I could and get my wife to type them out for me at home. This meant I often ended up undercharging because I'd forgotten some detail or other. Now, for the first time in my life, I can write neatly and spell confidently – and I am making more money. I wish the programme had been available 20 years ago!'

Bob, builder, 32

'When I did the assessments the second time, the lady at the centre told me how much better I had done. I thought, Yeah, yeah. Then I saw the computer printout from the balancing test – there it was on paper how much I had improved. Great!'

Todd, 11

The greatest improvement patterns are shown in those who have been very consistent in doing their exercises at home, twice a day, for around ten minutes each time.

'I got a bit lazy and fell behind in my charts and on the third visit it showed in my assessments – there's no cheating!'

Diane, 15

For some, the results are rapid and the programme may be completed in as little as nine months. In a few cases, others may need to continue up to 18 months. However, when the exercises are done regularly, the average programme seems to last for about 12 months. In Simon's case, he completed it in a rather rapid eight months.

'It is unbelievable that a year ago I was miserable – I couldn't see the point in going on, life was such a struggle. Today I feel like a new person, and it is all thanks to Dore Achievement Centres.'

Robbie, 32

THE RAPID CHANGE PHASE

We have noticed that some can experience a short period of increased emotional turbulence while in the early stages of a programme. This is not as unpleasant as it sounds, nor does it last long: it is merely a natural response to the rapid change or maturing that is occurring in the cerebellum. Some do not have this experience at all but those who do may feel:

- Some increase in moodiness or irritability
- A period of introspection (particularly in adults)
- A temporary period of forgetfulness with what would normally be an automatic task.

If they do occur, these emotional phases are temporary, lasting typically for only a few weeks, and once you know to expect them

they are easy to cope with and understand. In fact, they are quite like what happens in the 'terrible twos' or early teens. In both cases, these are periods of rapid cerebellar development so it is not surprising.

> *'I felt snappy and crabby with those around me and my wife was a bit surprised, but within a matter of days I was back to my normal self.'*
>
> Dan, 45

> *'For about a week my son had attitude and I was worried we were back to the way things had been before we started the programme. They had warned me at the centre he might feel this way, and I called them for reassurance. We carried on with the exercises as they said we should, and by the next visit he was happier and more confident than he had been before the moody period.'*
>
> Sally, Todd's mum

Chapter 14

HOW THIS PROGRAMME MIGHT MAKE YOU INTO A BETTER SPORTSPERSON

I should make it very clear that in the early days of the programme we were only trying to find a solution for dyslexia. Our aim was to discover a breakthrough treatment that could help people with their reading, writing and concentration ability, and at the time we did not think about the possible impact the programme might have on other areas like a person's overall co-ordination. It was not long, however, before stories about how the programme was making a huge difference to people's sporting ability began to appear.

You may remember our first two case studies, Simon Wheeler and Jamie Frances, from earlier in the book. The progress that both these boys made in terms of their sporting ability was absolutely astounding.

Jamie was our second guinea pig and started the same week as my daughter, Susie. He had suffered from low-self-esteem issues, partially because he was not good at sport; he really wanted to be able to play tennis with his older brothers, who were both

accomplished sportsmen, but he had great difficulty connecting the racket with the ball. Cutting a long story short, soon after he completed the programme, his sporting ability and self-esteem had improved so much that he was made class captain and later head boy. He is now an accomplished rower, the youngest qualified rowing coach in the county and also runs to a very high standard with one of the local athletics clubs.

Simon also saw some dramatic improvements. Before doing the programme, when he was 13, he already had a golf handicap of 26. By the time he had come through the course, this had reduced to 10. He has since gone on to play golf for his county and recently came second in the British Schoolboy Golf Competition.

We also had some amazing results in sport when we carried out the research project at Balsall Common School. You can read about these findings in Chapter 10 (pages 135–149), but in short the headmaster came to me one day and said that his soccer teams were filling up with students who had gone through the programme. What was particularly heart-warming about this was that previously many of these pupils had such poor co-ordination they could barely kick a ball. Suddenly, they were winning all sorts of sporting awards and gaining popularity because of their newfound skills.

I could barely contain my excitement at all these amazing results. Although we had focused on learning and attention issues, it seemed that many of the brain's other functions were also improved by the exercises. Stories kept coming in about how patients were suddenly seeing huge improvements in their sporting ability and our files were bursting to capacity with more and more anecdotes.

For example, one of our earliest trials was with a highly talented young gymnast called Rose Meredith, who was at the

time ranked tenth in the country for her age. Her parents suggested that she went through the programme because, despite obvious intelligence, she did not find reading and writing as easy as she would have liked, and they hoped we could help. When Rose was doing the balance test required before she could start the programme, we had assumed that because of her gymnastic training she would get first-rate balance results. After all, she was training for four hours every night of the week. When the results came through, however, we could see there were a few very distinct, but important areas we felt we could improve in her balance development. In fact, the research therapist who tested Rose was puzzled as to how she could possibly have managed to do so well in some routines, including juggling. Rose was very suspicious that the therapist had been talking to her coach because she had pointed out exactly the areas where she could do with help.

So Rose started to do the programme and, one night, after she had been doing the exercises for a number of weeks, her dad heard a scream coming from his daughter's room. He ran up the stairs and burst open the door, fearing something dreadful had happened, only to find that Rose had a huge smile on her face and she was juggling effortlessly for the first time in her life. Previously, she had tried on countless occasions to do this and had ended up throwing her gymnastic batons down in utter frustration. Suddenly, something seemed to have clicked in her head and remarkably the automaticity required for her to juggle had kicked in. For Rose, this was a major breakthrough and it paved the way for another amazing achievement: only a few months later, she won the National Pairs Gymnastic Championship. Today, Rose is thoroughly enjoying studying at university and is showing her real potential.

The famous Scottish rugby star, Kenny Logan, is another example of someone who noticed a significant improvement in his already wonderful sporting skills. When he started on the programme, Kenny had been playing at the highest level of rugby for over ten years. He had come because he wanted to improve his reading and writing, but by the end of the course he was shocked to find that he was playing the best rugby of his life. Kenny experienced so many positive benefits that, like so many others, he has become passionate about helping to spread the message that others do not need to face the trauma he did as he struggled through school life. His efforts to help others are tireless and he has personally influenced thousands of young people to undertake what has proven to be a life-changing experience for them, too.

THE SCIENCE BEHIND THE IMPACT ON SPORTING SKILLS

Elite sportspeople develop their skills initially through a genetic predisposition to be skilful, fit and focused. The perfect combination to create an elite athlete would be good genes to allow better physical development and fitness, perfect and complete neurological development to enable skill learning and, finally, those personality traits that make someone focus – and remain focused – on winning.

But not all athletes share the same traits. Some have the natural physical development and fitness levels due to physiological advantages; some develop skills very easily; others get there by being the most focused and determined personalities. The supreme athlete will have all of these traits. Some of these advantages are purely genetically determined and, until we develop genetic engineering to its highest level or perhaps legalise cloning, this cannot be altered. Mental effort and

focus is also a reflection of personality that can be genetically determined but it is much more influenced by environmental factors. Often focus and determination can come from early-life experiences. To nurture these traits, good coaching and mentoring are vital and top sportsmen rely heavily on sports psychologists to help maintain their focus and determination.

Physical build – especially height – is genetically determined, but build can also be influenced by diet and training methods. The same applies to fitness. It is well known that muscle physiology is genetically determined and many of the top athletes have advantages due to this in terms of power, metabolism and stamina. Once again, good training can have a profound effect on fitness levels, which, with the exception of the sports requiring the most endurance can compensate fully for any shortfall in genetic gifts. However, up until now, little has been done to address the neurological advantages that we now appreciate could help tremendously.

Where high levels of skill are required to achieve, many top athletes and sportspeople usually succeed due to their ability to learn and automatise skills to the point of almost subconscious ability. This type of learning is termed procedural. With practice, skills are fine-tuned and enhanced to a point of automaticity, which allows a sportsman to reproduce manoeuvres very precisely. Depending on the complexity of the skill (i.e. the number of practices required to make that skill automatic), skilled manoeuvres take differing amounts of time to perfect. Some take thousands or even tens of thousands of repetitions to do this.

When one considers elite sports stars, despite their having practised for years, even at their level there are still marked differences in their level of ability. Why can't every footballer bend the ball like Beckham, read the game like Gascoigne or have the

footwork skills of Zidane? The reason lies in the neurological mechanisms whereby skills are learned and automated to allow repeated accuracy and improving abilities to adjust to differing conditions. This requires the development of both thinking brain (cerebral cortex) and, more importantly, the cerebellum (hindbrain). The thinking brain alone can develop skill but at such a poor rate of improvement that it takes much, much longer and will never become automatic or elite.

If you want to be really scientific, you can calculate the number of repetitions (X) needed to learn a given skill if the area of the cerebellum responsible for learning that skill is not completely developed. The formula is

$$X = y_x\sqrt{y}$$

where y is the typical number of repetitions needed to learn a skill when the cerebellum is fully developed. So, for simple skills like doing up buttons – for example, it might take 25 attempts to learn to do this. If cerebellar function is poor, it takes 25 multiplied by the square root of 25 (i.e. 5), which is 125 times. With some patience, this is easily achievable. However, if one considers a complex skill, then this can take very much longer. For example, if it takes 900 attempts to learn a skill to perfection, if the cerebellar function responsible for that type of skill was poor, this might take 900 x the square root of 900 (30), which is 27,000 repetition. Unless someone is incredibly determined, they are very unlikely to practise it that many times!

The reason for this is that the brain alone is not equipped to develop these elite motor skills. Despite its power, the thinking brain works too slowly to enable the control of the rapid and fine adjustments to movement and thus allow the retention of these

very precise programmes of skill. What would happen if we could somehow train the cerebellum to improve its function to enable a more rapid development of skills and enhance those already learned skills to get to an even higher level of performance and automaticity? The answer would be an overall enhanced level of skill and performance allowing better automatisation and thus release working memory to be available for other tasks. This would enable sportsmen to read the game, follow team strategies better and allow all players to play as a team and less as individually skilled entities. We believe this programme can achieve this.

Using sophisticated neuro-physiological tests and examinations we are able to assess cerebellar function and to use a precise and personalised programme of stimulatory exercises to enhance cerebellar function for the most elite athletes. Dore has already published peer-reviewed research on the effectiveness of these programmes in schools with those pupils who previously were showing significant cerebellar under-functioning. Many of these pupils went on to show huge academic gains and also huge gains in sporting ability. A number of elite sportspeople have also been on our programme and noticed the ability to improve existing skills, develop new skills that they found difficult to do before and to automatise skills better, making it easier to read the game and concentrate right to the end of it.

Since then, we have developed more highly specific and stimulatory exercises for elite sportspeople. The programme consists of a number of exercises that, through intense stimulation of the different parts of the vestibular system, permanently improve the cerebellar function. The result is a more automatic control of the body during movement. There is improved ability to control movement change, precise use of

visual reflexes that in turn create even better ball skills through more precise determination of ball flight. Overall, these exercises will allow:

- Faster acquisition of new skills
- Automatisation and consistency in the use of acquired skills
- Increased spatial awareness, which in turn gives a greater ability to judge the game and anticipate moves
- Better co-ordination of movement and change of movement at speed (faster reactions and timing)
- Precise visual reflexes while moving to make more precise judgements of ball flight and timing
- Ability to focus for the whole game (attention skills are sustained as well, as the brain gets less tired by processing less unautomatised skills)
- Better self-esteem — more likely to be positive and have 'a winner's attitude'
- Better control of frustration and temper (enhances emotional control).

Elite sportspeople are able to perform at the highest level. To move to an even higher level requires only an improvement of a few per cent.

Chapter 15

FOUR SUCCESS STORIES

REBECCA WATTS (11 YEARS) BY LORA WATTS

Rebecca Watts was a shy girl with few friends and no confidence. She found reading and writing extremely difficult and got so frustrated and depressed that she even told her mother, 'Heaven may be a better place than here because I wouldn't have to go to school every day.' She came to Dore in Southampton in October 2002.

I first suspected Rebecca might have problems when she was seven and I read her bedtime stories. I would go over and over simple rhymes like 'Humpty Dumpty' and she just couldn't grasp them. I was a bit worried so my husband and I decided to have her eyes and ears tested, but the results showed she was perfectly healthy and that she just was not interested in books.

However, when she started school I noticed that she was becoming increasingly unhappy. She hated reading and would only read when she had to at school, never at home. After a

couple of years, Rebecca's teachers realised she could barely read – up to that point she had been fooling them by guessing the captions beneath the pictures in her books. Unfortunately, by the time they had noticed this, she was already miles behind in her studies. They put her on an intensive reading course and insisted hard work was all she needed to catch up but no amount of effort seemed to do the trick.

Rebecca also had other problems that had begun to show themselves. She was having real difficulty with her handwriting, which must have looked like a foreign language to anyone else reading it. She also continued to have problems retaining information, whether it was nursery rhymes or dance steps and sequences; even learning to tell the time was a real problem.

Around this time, I started to think to myself that Rebecca must be dyslexic. I myself had struggled with dyslexia when I was younger and seeing all the problems that Rebecca was going through started to set the alarm bells ringing. I was not concerned about making Rebecca an academic star – I just wanted her to be happy. In the end, we decided to move her to another school. This proved to be a worthless move as she was put into a special-needs section of her new class and became an instant target for bullies and name-calling.

She would regularly come to me in tears and ask if she could change schools. She was actually a twin but I miscarried during the pregnancy. Rebecca started saying maybe it would be better for her to join her twin – it was so painful to hear her talk like that.

As Rebecca became more and more frustrated, she became full of emotional rage; she would become very tired and despondent, and draw dark and morbid pictures that were extremely worrying. She felt like she was being treated like an idiot at school. She was

seven and a half and they were giving her the alphabet to learn! She would complain that she was not stupid and say she knew the alphabet, but just couldn't put the letters together to make words and sentences.

I took Rebecca to see an educational psychologist. Tests showed that there were learning problems and the final report stated that Rebecca was definitely dyslexic. The problem was I did not know what to do next. Thankfully, not long after, a relative phoned me and told me she had seen a television programme about a new treatment for dyslexia that was supposedly working miracles.

I went to the Dore Achievement Centre headquarters in Kenilworth where Rebecca's writing, hearing, eyesight, balance and co-ordination were assessed. Over four hours, she was given written tests, a maths exam, reading tests and an interview by a child psychologist. Some people might think the cost of the treatment is expensive, but I would have been prepared to pay double just to see Rebecca happy.

Following her assessment, Rebecca was prescribed an individualised exercise programme to carry out at home twice a day. She carried out the fun-to-do exercises every day and, although sometimes it was tempting not to do them, with my support she kept them up. Every six weeks, Rebecca returned to the centre for testing to see how much she had improved and was given her next set of exercises.

At first, I thought some of the exercises she was doing were bonkers. She would have to do things like standing on one leg for 30 seconds and concentrate on keeping still. There was another one that involved sitting on an exercise ball and staying balanced. She had to do these exercises twice a day, but we were desperate, so we decided to give it a chance. However, it was not long before

we began to see incredible changes. First of all, her balance improved and she was suddenly able to do things like rollerblading down the drive. But it was not just her balance that improved. Suddenly, she was able to read signposts and she would blurt out things as we drove around.

As she went through the programme, the exercises became tougher. For example, she would have to close her eyes and stand on one leg while tossing a beanbag from one hand to the other. But the effects the exercises were having were astounding. Processing thoughts, her reading and writing all started to become much easier for her. Before she had done the programme, it would take her about half an hour to complete a paragraph, suddenly she could write a whole page in that time. The crowning glory came when she gained her silver handwriting certificate. She was so thrilled and, as her ability grew, so did her confidence. Quite simply she was a much happier child.

She was, by that point, approaching her last few weeks at junior school and she was expecting to get one Grade II and two Grade III passes in her SATs (Statutory Assessment Tests). Instead, she stunned teachers by getting three Grade IV results.

I realise it sounds too good to be true; I needed proof like anybody else but I have seen it work firsthand and the change in Rebecca has been astounding, nothing short of a miracle! It is like having a new daughter, a new Rebecca. I do not go through the day dreading hearing her crying any more. The programme has transformed our lives and all it took was five minutes of exercises every night. The difference to my daughter is amazing. She now looks at herself as a worthy human being who has credibility amongst her peers. She is brimming with a newfound confidence and self-belief.

I now have a happy child who paints pictures full of colour;

she is happy and laughs a lot – the way most 11-year-olds should – it's just great.

SAM LINDLEY (TEN YEARS) BY SARA LINDLEY

This is the story of how a little boy who could hardly write his own name went on to be runner-up in a national writing competition.

I had always known there was a possibility that Sam was dyslexic because it ran in the family. My husband and his father had always had reading problems and my sister-in-law's two sons both had recognised dyslexia. So, with all the boys in the family suffering from the condition, the chances that Sam would somehow escape from it were not good.

Sam was seven when he came to me one day and said he did not want to go to school any more. I knew my fears had been realised and it broke my heart. I asked him why and he said he couldn't do the maths any more and he couldn't read or write properly.

The teachers at school were very surprised by this because Sam had a very good vocabulary and they assumed he would be able to write it all down. But the fact was he couldn't put pen to paper and doing so just made him tired and frustrated. He had huge difficulties with letters and would often reverse them and write them the wrong way around. He had a particular problem with 'S' and even found it tricky to write his own name. 'D' and 'B' also gave him trouble because they looked very similar, as did 'P' and 'Q'. He would also get numbers muddled up so that, if he wanted to write '13', he would actually put down '31'.

Reading was also a nightmare and he could only read one or two lines before he would start to get upset. The tragedy of this was that he loved books. He loved it when people read to him and

he was a big fan of Roald Dahl. But, when he had to pick up a book himself, it was a different story. It was so sad for him watching all his friends enjoying reading while he struggled to get through much easier books.

Sam had always had very poor co-ordination and was not very good at sports. I remember one day we had to teach him how to run because he couldn't work out how to move his arms in time with his legs. It was particularly embarrassing for him because our younger son was able to hurtle up and down the drive without any problems. In contrast, Sam's arms and legs were all over the place. On another occasion, Sam was playing with a swingball and was having problems hitting the ball with his bat. He managed to hit about ten balls in a row, but gave up and watched as his brother got a score of 150. He would never throw an absolute temper tantrum but you could see he was getting frustrated and it was sapping away at his confidence.

When we realised he was dyslexic, we looked into sending him to the Dyslexia Foundation to be assessed. As I was a primary school teacher, I was also prepared to give him the extra help he needed to catch up. Purely by coincidence, while we were trying to work out how we could best help our son, the Trevor McDonald programme went out and that is how we found out about Dore.

My husband and I were very impressed by what we saw. We could see the logic in the programme and we loved the fact it was a non-invasive treatment. There was no way we were going to have our son taking all sorts of different drugs, which could harm him. Having him do exercises every day, therefore, seemed a much better option.

When we went to the Dore Centre, Sam was tested to see if he was dyslexic. The assessment said that he had mild dyslexia. The tests were very thorough and ranged from eye-tracking tests and

balancing tests to spelling words. It was actually a great relief to have it confirmed that Sam had a learning difficulty. However, I did suspect that his problem might be worse than the results had shown. The reason his symptoms were not more apparent was probably because he had a high IQ, which had helped him develop ways of masking the problem. As my background was in teaching, the aid I had given him may also have stopped him from getting a lower score. Nevertheless, the problems he faced were not mild to him and he even wrote his name wrong on the test paper.

The original exercises he was given involved beanbags, wobble boards and a big ball. I remember one of the first exercises involved standing on one leg, throwing a beanbag in the air and trying to catch it in his other hand while reciting his two times table. He couldn't do it and he fell over. Trying to remember how to do all those things at once was really tough for him. As soon as he had to think about something else, he would completely lose his co-ordination. I must admit at that early stage I couldn't imagine what on earth any of this had to do with his reading or his writing. It certainly was not a small commitment, and some tears were shed. I could see how people might find it hard to keep up the routine. However, Sam was determined and thankfully he stuck at it.

It took about 12 weeks before we began to notice very slight changes in Sam. It was little things like being able to catch the beanbag without dropping it. We also noticed his co-ordination was getting better and he did not seem quite as tired as he had been before. The real improvement we noticed was in his reading. There was never a single dramatic 'hey presto!' moment, but it was obvious he was progressing. One day, he read a whole book to me. It was not an easy book and it was an absolutely fantastic

moment. I told him to go and show his dad, but by that point he was tiring and the second time through was not quite as good. Even so, this was a pivotal moment and a very proud moment for me. I could see how much he had enjoyed reading it and how his confidence was growing. He was also really pleased with himself; he had always adored books and loved them being read to him. Now, for the first time, he was beginning to read them all the way through to himself.

Now he has a collection of Roald Dahl and Alex Rider books that he adores and reading has become less of a problem and more of a passion. He continually surprises his teachers with his progress. The last time I spoke to his teacher, Sam was six months above his reading age. He'd always been well below his reading age before so this was a real triumph. Teachers still say that he has to concentrate hard to learn a new skill but, once he has learned the technique, it sticks in his head. Homework is no longer a chore for him. When he comes home from school, he is more than happy to do it.

In sport, too, there were some big changes. He used to play football and was a defender. This position suited him as he had time to see people running at him and could decide how to react. When it came to on-the-spot decision making, like many people with dyslexia he had problems and would not be so good. Now it is totally different. When he comes home from school, he often tells us he was the best player on the team. While this may not be true, it is beautiful to hear him say it, to see that he has developed self-belief.

There was a nationwide competition around the 40th anniversary of the *Charlie and the Chocolate Factory* book by Roald Dahl. Contestants were asked to invent a new naughty child character for the book. Over the summer, Sam wrote a description

of a character and drew a picture to accompany it. Sam invented 'Warty Walter Mouthwater' and, keeping to the 100-word limit, described who he was. It really illustrated to me how much his thought process had come on since doing the programme. This is what he wrote:

Warty Walter Mouthwater
Loves cheese. He eats so much that fat, ugly mouldy warts burst out from the tip of his nose to the end of his toes. He has smelly, cheesy breath and a green hairy tongue. Because of the way he looks and smells, people run away from the pong. He doesn't like chocolate so he decides to change chocolate history.

The perfect chocolate for his scam was the chocolate mice because, of course, mice like cheese. Walter creeps away from the tour and from his emergency stash he threw some cheese into the chocolate mice-mixing tank. The cheese sank, bubbling into the mixture.

Yellowy brown, cheesy chocolate mice appeared, took one whiff of Walter and sprang to life. They leapt onto Walter and dragged him off into their giant mouse hole. Walter only returned when all of his warts were nibbled away and his cheesy smell had gone.

The day came when the results were announced. Sam was so disappointed that he hadn't won. However, just a short time later, we heard that he was one of the runners-up. His actual picture was assessed by Quentin Blake himself, who was one of Sam's heroes, and he was sent a selection of Roald Dahl books. I was so pleased for him. He had been working exceptionally hard at school and it was great to see him get a reward. Before the

programme, Sam wouldn't have thought a pile of books was any sort of prize at all unless I said I would read them to him. Now he can read a book in one go and is the happiest he has ever been.

On Sam's final day at the centre, we bumped into a man who I instantly recognised as Wynford Dore. I was so pleased to be able to thank him for what his treatment had done for my son. We were on our way to give his equipment back (Sam's wobble board, etc.) and Wynford turned to Sam and asked, 'Would you like to keep it?' to which he responded, 'Yes, please.' It was just like the story of Willy Wonka and it was the dream way to end the course.

STUART JONES (15) BY ELAINE JONES

Stuart Jones was singled out as a troublemaker by his teachers. After doing the programme, he has gone from being a problem child to being a golden boy.

The worst day I ever experienced was when I was called into Stuart's school and had to listen to criticism after criticism about my son's bad behaviour. Stuart was 12 at the time and by that point I was already used to hearing complaints from his teachers about how he would get up and walk around in the middle of a lesson, or whisper to his friends. In fact, it seemed like I was going up to his school almost every week because he had landed himself in some sort of trouble. Whether it was a fight in the playground or an incident in the classroom, Stuart somehow seemed to be involved and sometimes I felt like his teachers had my number on speed dial.

On this one particular occasion, however, the situation was very different. Both Stuart's father and I had been asked to attend a meeting along with our son to discuss his progress. Normally, when we had been summoned to a meeting in the past there had

been just a few of us, but this time the room was full of people. The headmaster was there, a learning support teacher, a special-needs teacher and Stuart's own teacher were all in the room. It was quite an intimidating situation and things only got worse. Before the meeting got started, I pleaded with them, 'Please tell me some positive things, do not just criticise him,' but my request fell on deaf ears.

Everything they had to say was negative and it turned out that the reason they had called the meeting was they did not want to let Stuart go on the school history trip. They said he was obviously in a depression and his behaviour was too disruptive to risk taking him away with the school. Stuart just started to cry and cry, and I turned to the headmaster and said, 'You have children! Would you let four adults go on at your child like this?' I'd had enough and I was not going to sit there and let my son be bullied. However, at the same time, I knew we had a problem and I did not know what to do about it.

The fact was Stuart *was* in a depression. He was not the happy-go-lucky boy he had once been. Since he had started high school, there had been a big change in his attitude. The turning point came when one day in English his teacher asked him to read out loud to the class and he refused to do it. From that moment on, the other kids started to notice there was something different about him and would pick on him and call him names. He got more and more frustrated because he couldn't do certain things as easily as his friends could. His reading was laboured and slow, and he never picked up a book. He also had problems with writing and often you couldn't make out what he had written because of his terrible spelling. His vocabulary was also bad and he had great trouble writing paragraphs. Sometimes he would try really hard, but he couldn't do it and would end up panicking

about everything. By Christmas, he had really sunk into a bad depression and he did not want to eat or do anything.

Throughout high school, things had got progressively worse. There were several big incidents in the school, which almost resulted in his suspension. I used to always hear complaints that Stuart was a name-caller. This was hard to believe because he was always so polite at home. When I asked him why he had been calling other people names, he told me that he was just responding to being called 'thicko' or 'stupid'. I know two wrongs do not make a right, but I was relieved to hear that he was only standing up for himself and not a bully. I am not condoning his behaviour, but in the end, if you have to put up with insults all day, every day, it is hard not to react.

He had already been assessed as having dyslexia and desperately needed help, but his school was very reluctant to give him the extra time he needed. As far as they were concerned, he was lazy and just needed to work harder. In the end, thanks to the support of a few very kind teachers, he was allowed to have a reader in his exams. All of a sudden, his marks went up. It was a small victory; I knew Stuart had the potential to do better than the marks he had been getting. However, his achievement was tainted by the fact that he had needed a reader; he wouldn't be able to get this sort of help in real life. We had already sent him to tutors, had him tested and had bought him many handbooks to help him read, but he hadn't improved. Before I found out about the programme, I was at my wits' end.

I was told about the programme after Stuart had failed an exam to be a referee. He had always been very good at sport – in fact, he was talent-spotted by Oxford United when he was eight and he wanted to be a referee. When he failed the test, I can honestly say I'd never seen him looking so miserable. A friend of mine, whose

daughter had been on the programme, told me all about how it had transformed her life and how she was excelling in her studies. When I told Stuart about it, he did not need a lot of convincing that it might be worth doing. As far as he was concerned, anything that would help him pass his exam was worth a shot.

When we were at the clinic waiting to see the Dore specialist, I turned to Stuart and asked, 'Are you sure you are going to give this your full attention? Because I am not going to spend all this money for you to give up in a couple of days.' He told me he really wanted to do it. Clearly, he was as desperate as I was for his life to change.

There is no other word to describe the change in Stuart but amazing. I had noticed his writing had got better after just a few months on the programme. In English, for example, he used to always struggle to write just a few paragraphs for his homework, and that was on a good day. Suddenly, he was writing three or four pages and we were forcing him to do it. He started coming home every day from school with a new determination and would sit at his desk and just pour words out on to the pages.

After five months of doing his exercises, it was time for him to sit his referee exam again. The results speak for themselves. He got 59 out of 60 for his oral examination and for his written he had got 29 out of 40. Bearing in mind he did not have a reader or any help at all, these results were incredible. When he came out of the exam, he said to me, 'Mum, the programme is working because I read every question myself.' To hear my child say that is absolutely amazing.

He is now doing a diploma in sport and has already got two A*s and two As. He stays behind late after school to work on his biology and, although he was predicted to get an E in his English GCSE, he has already got a B for his *Macbeth* coursework.

In every aspect of his life, he has just got stronger and stronger. These days I do not have to spend every five minutes being worried about the school calling me up. In fact, the last time they called me, it was because he had accidentally smashed a window with a football. I was not pleased about it but it was much better than being called up because he had smacked someone over the head. His sporting ability has also seen huge improvements. If you ask anybody in the area where I live, 'Who is Stuart Jones?' they will say that he is the best goalie in the town. It is true that he has always been a keen sportsman, but before the programme he always seemed a little bit inward. He lacked confidence and would be afraid to shout things out in case people would think what he said was stupid. Now his interpersonal skills are brilliant and he directs the field of play. If you watch him on Sunday, all the other dads will say things like, 'Cor, look how he reads the game! Look how he talks to his teammates!' I am very proud because I never thought it would get to this stage.

One of the proudest moments happened during a sports match. Stuart was playing shot put for his school and was up against quite fierce competition. He was lying in third place when one of his competitors started to boast that Stuart should give up because he was not going to win. Stuart gave it his all and ended up throwing the furthest distance. The other boy was furious and started saying all sorts of rude things, but Stuart just walked away, unaffected. He even helped the teacher measure the distance of the throws. After he had won the medal, one of the teachers from the other school said Stuart was the politest 14-year-old she had ever met.

The following day, when Stuart went to school, the headmaster called him to his office. The first thing that Stuart said was, 'I haven't done anything wrong today.'

To this, the headmaster replied, 'I have just had a call from a teacher at another school. She says she was so proud of you for how well you represented your school and that we should be proud of you, too.'

Stuart responded, 'The trouble is, Sir, that you had put a label on me. Like my mum says, you should never judge a book by its cover, you should have a look inside. If you had looked at me for what I am before, you would have always known I was a nice person.'

Dyslexia is no longer something that my son is embarrassed about. He is not afraid to tell people about the exercises he did. The way he sees it, dyslexia is just a problem he overcame. Before, however, it was a different story. He had been ashamed and had tried to hide it. In the end, he just became deeply frustrated and depressed. If people learn anything from his story, I hope that the most important thing is coming to terms with dyslexia because that is the only way you will get help.

TINA BOGGET'S STORY (38)
'I couldn't understand why God had made life so hard for me and why I couldn't be normal like everyone else.'

It was when I was little that I knew I was different from other children. I was put in a class for children with special needs, but it was when I got older that I started to feel the effect that dyslexia had on me. I always felt alone and that people did not like me. In the playground, I did not fit, or if I did it wouldn't be long before I felt left out by my friends; I would just stand and watch.

I was very moody and would cry a lot. I always played with the children that were dropouts, but I now know that they probably had dyslexia like me. As I got older, life got harder because I

realised that I was different. I left school and got a job in a factory, but I only got that because a friend of mine had turned it down. I must admit that I picked the job up very quickly. I was there for five years and was quite happy. I had a fall-out with another woman and I had to leave because I always worried about what she was telling other people; I always need people to like me.

From that factory, I went to work at a company called C.I. Caravans. I was there for two years and was quite happy at first. There was a girl who really got to me. She was OK at first, but when we fell out she made my life hell. I wanted to hit her, but the men I worked with stopped me and said that she was not worth it. My nerves got so bad that I couldn't even go to the toilet all day. My day started at 7.30am and did not finish until 5.00 pm, so you can imagine how hard it could be for me some days. She got her comeuppance, as she was made redundant, which really made my day.

Not long after that, I met my husband, Paul, and I left the factory to live with him in Melton Mowbray. I did not have much luck when it came to men. I found it very hard to communicate, but Paul was different – he helped me a lot. When you have dyslexia, you find it very hard to express your feelings and you hold a lot in.

I found it very frustrating because I had always wanted to own my own business, but I did not know where to start. I had my first child, a little girl called Jennifer, but, as time went on, I found that I did not have much patience with her. I would sometimes get angry with her when she did not do as she was told. I was very emotional and never seemed to be on an even scale, always up and down.

As I got older, I started to get depressed. I had my second child, Lisa, who was very hard work. She slept through the night

from an early age, but she wouldn't go to other people. Every time I left the room without her, she would scream or cry. She was about three years old when I had a breakdown and I did not know where my life was going. I couldn't understand why God had made life so hard for me and why I couldn't be normal like everyone else. I went to college to see if there was any help for me and I met a lady who tested me for dyslexia.

When she told me that I did have dyslexia, I could have cried. I knew that there was something wrong but, when a name is put to the problem, it is hard to accept. I went home and told Paul. He tried to get me to look at all the things I had done with my life and the things that I had achieved. He did not know what I felt inside. I had become very clever at covering up my dyslexia by putting on a good front so people never knew. After being told about the dyslexia, I began to accept it, but it took a good year to come to terms with it. However, I still had problems. I worked at a play school and trying to remember the children's names was a nightmare.

I also did cleaning and selling clothes at a car boot sale. From the car boot sales I started doing clothes parties and that was when I found out that what I was good at: selling. So I opened a shop selling second-hand clothes. This went so well that I now sell new clothes. My ambition is to sell designer clothes.

I had been out walking my dog, Bobby, and when I came home the TV programme *Tonight* starring Trevor McDonald was just about to start. The programme topic was about dyslexia. I couldn't believe my ears; what I was hearing was that there was possibly a cure for dyslexia. I sat down and cried; my dream had come true at last. I was determined that I was going to be the first in the queue for treatment. I was so excited I rang my mum and said that they might have found a cure for dyslexia but I do not

think that she knew how much I had suffered throughout my life. When Paul came home, I made him sit down and watch the programme, which I had videoed. At first, I did not think that we could be able to afford it, but Paul said that he would work overtime to pay for the treatment, as he knew how much it meant to me.

My first appointment was on 26 June 2002. I went to the Dore Centre in Bedford, where I was tested for dyslexia. The doctor confirmed that I did have dyslexia and the treatment that they offered could help. I started the exercises straight away and, within one week, I had seen a difference in me. I was reading the newspaper one day and it suddenly hit me that I actually read the whole story and not just the headline. Before, I would get bored with it and push it away. As the weeks went by, I became more confident and dealt with problems. I did not feel guilty about things I said, whereas before I would have worried. I was a lot calmer and more relaxed, too. I can now deal with problems and move on.

My reading went from nothing to fluent, as if I'd been doing it all my life. It is nice to be able to read to my two girls at bedtime and help them with their homework. Jennifer used to help me spell, but now it is me helping her. The dyslexia exercises have helped me move on in my life. I have enrolled for a computer course and a counselling course, something I thought that I would never do. I had to give a talk about how the dyslexia treatment has helped me to a group of approximately 200 people. I stood up and told the people how having done the course had changed my life.

The proudest moment was when my two girls and I were travelling home from my mum's and Lisa wanted to do some spellings. Jennifer said that she'd do them with Lisa, but Lisa

turned round and said, 'I want my mum to do them because you might get them wrong.' You can imagine how proud that made me feel. I always tell people about my dyslexia and how the treatment has worked. I am so proud of myself.

When I started doing the exercises, the change was gradual. I'd be sitting reading and, when I came to a word that I did not know, I found that I could break it down and put it together and make sense of it. The first word I broke down was 'triumphantly' and I really surprised myself that I could do it. Then I noticed that my reading was more fluent and not broken. I found that I locked on to words that were there and read them all. Before I would have lost my place and would miss words out and put words in that were not there at all.

Within three days of doing the exercises, I noticed that I was walking taller and holding my head up instead of looking at the ground. Some of my friends would ask me if I'd lost weight as I held myself up better. I used to have a problem with my right foot and I couldn't wear a pair of high-heeled shoes. If I did, my foot would be in so much pain within ten minutes of wearing them. Since doing the exercises, my posture has straightened and is taking the weight off my right foot so the pain has gone. It is so nice to be able to put on a dress with a pair of high-heeled shoes instead of wearing flat shoes and feeling frumpy.

I also noticed I was able to do certain things that I had not been able to do before. I can now swim a full length of front crawl and breaststroke, and can get the breathing right. Before, I would only do a few strokes before choking; now I am up and down the pool like a fish.

I am a lot more relaxed when it comes to driving. Before, if I did not know where I was going, I would panic and hold on to the steering wheel for dear life and be really tense. Now I do not panic

and I relax when I am driving. One day my husband and I got lost in Leeds and my husband was having kittens. I turned round to him and said, 'You should be doing my exercises, dear!'

This one I cannot believe: I used to hate cooking and would do anything to get out of it. It used to be anything out of the freezer, packet or tin. Once I bought a cake mix to make. All I had to do was to add water and shake, but it did not get baked. I now enjoy cooking and do some nice dinners. My girls mark me out of 10.

I am now able to sort out my own problems on the phone when it is to do with my own business. Before, I would get Paul to sort it out for me. I am finding that I understand things better and pick things up quicker.

My personality has changed as well. I am not so moody any more; I get on so much better with my oldest daughter, whereas before we would be at each other's throat. She can see a lot of change in me. There's no more shouting in the morning when getting ready for school; I do not get irritable over little things any more. I seem to have a lot more patience and seem to be more laidback. Before, I would put up a front and let people know I was not going to be messed with. I am very proud about the way I handle problems now with other people. I do not fly off the handle and jump down their throats any more. I deal with the problems and do not feel guilty about what I have said. Before, I would worry about what I had said. My husband's brother, Mark, said that I have gone from being a cub to a lioness in dealing with problems. I can now say 'no' to people and to things that I do not want to do. Before I would say 'yes' just to keep the peace.

This may sound a bit hard but I have a nice group of friends now. Before, I had friends who all had problems, which drained me of energy. I do not rush to help people so much now because

I realise that you have to look after yourself. I had some friends round for drinks and, when they got up to leave, my friend Dot went to cuddle me. It felt the most natural thing to do. If anyone had come near me before, I would have tensed up and done anything to get out of cuddling people.

I remember people's names now, which is nice because I have my own shop and deal with a lot of people. Many of these have become friends so it is nice to be able to remember their names as well as their faces. I have been to my husband's works Christmas party for the last four years and this year was the first time that I felt that I fitted in. Before, I felt inferior to the other women and thought that they looked down their noses at me. Dyslexia can make you feel like this, as though you do not fit in. This was the first time since doing the exercises that I felt as though I did fit in and did not feel inferior.

I am so much happier with my life now. I feel normal at last; I feel as though I belong now when talking to other people. I now say that I *had* dyslexia – I do not class myself as being dyslexic any more.

Chapter 16

LOOKING TO THE FUTURE

My dream has always been to get the much-needed help that this programme provides to everyone, regardless of whether or not they can afford it. Ultimately, this means lots of things:

- It must be very affordable, which means that governments must ultimately provide it for those who cannot afford it
- It means that it must be available in many countries and that means in many languages
- It means that we have to do even more research to measure the achievement with a wider range of symptoms than we have already measured
- It means that educationalists need to be educated so that they fully understand what causes learning difficulties, what corrects the issues and how to understand the children affected
- It means that schools everywhere must screen all pupils to identify who may have developmental issues within the cerebellum and are thus not achieving their full potential.

This vision has governed everything we have ever tried to do, and everything we continue doing. It has been a long, hard slog, but then we are trying to cause a paradigm shift and I guess that is not supposed to be easy.

GOING GLOBAL

While it is actually getting easier for us to open new centres now, I personally will not have the time or the resources to open centres everywhere they are needed. Thus, I predict we will need to develop partnerships around the world, but only with those organisations that are passionate about helping people with learning and attention problems. I have no intention at all of working with those whose only ambition is to make huge amounts of money. Of course, any organisation we work with has to be properly run on a sound basis. It has to be efficient, it has to have good-quality control, it has to have good management and good motivation. But one of the key requirements is that it must also be absolutely sincere in its determination to help folk who have learning issues. Fortunately, there are a number of organisations like this around and I have been overwhelmed by the offers of help. These have often come from the influential people whose children have been dramatically helped by going on the programme.

The reason we went to Australia, New Zealand and America was to prove that we could deliver the product safely abroad – that we could support it, train people and get the IT communications working, and so on. We have done that, and at the same time we have managed to get some very influential key supporters in these countries that have become powerful advocates for the programme.

We have also shown that the programme can transcend

language barriers. When we developed our sophisticated software, we knew that it was vital that one day we would be able to translate it into different languages. Thanks to this, we have already been able to open a centre in Taiwan, delivering the exercises in Chinese. Well, we thought we'd pick an easy second language to have a go at first! Before long, we will be announcing the rollout into Spain. Other languages will quickly follow after that, I suspect. Our first venture in Africa opens this year, thanks to a wonderful partner we now have in Durban. And why is she so keen to be involved? Her own granddaughter's life has already been changed wonderfully. She doesn't want others in her area to have to make that long flight to England every six weeks to get the same help.

We have thus laid a foundation to enable delivery into many other countries. Every day I am approached by a new person or organisation who has seen the need and probably seen the potential of the programme, too. Our next challenge is to have a structured plan to get the programme to every corner of the world.

MAKING THE PROGRAMME AFFORDABLE

The strategy that has always driven me is that the programme should be available to everyone. As I come from a working-class background myself, I do know that money for such things does not come easily. Paying for the programme for a child in the family is comparable to some family holidays, or upgrading your car. The main difference is that what you are actually paying for is the chance to transform someone's life permanently.

Having said this, it makes me feel incredibly sad to know that there are some people out there who, for one reason or another, will not be able to afford the cost themselves. My hope has always been that governments will one day help provide the programme

for all people in need. In the town of Parkes in Australia this is exactly what is happening, but at this time only there. Sadly, it is likely that the rest of the world will take a while to follow their excellent example. However, there are now the earliest signs that the Establishment is just beginning to understand the economic, social and human implications of the programme.

HOME SUPPORT

One of our next challenges is to make the programme even easier so that those without support at home can do it. Now, when someone does the exercise programme, it is better if an adult is there to help and make sure they do the exercises properly. In supportive families, this is relatively easy to do, but, sadly, there are an awful lot of children and adults out there who would not have the much-needed help. To overcome this problem, we are working on a number of exciting motivational and monitoring tools that we believe will make this whole process happen more independently of external emotional support and encouragement.

TACKLING OTHER CONDITIONS

We are impatient to start researching the ways these theories and exercise programmes may be developed further and be used to help people with other neurological conditions; autism, for example. Not only this, but we also want to look at ways of helping other physiological disabilities and emotional difficulties, such as depression, anorexia and possibly other conditions.

Why do we want to do this? Simply because we have noticed that many of our patients, including Susie, display other psychiatric conditions and other neurologically related symptoms besides just having reading and attention problems. Once we have mended their basic physiological problem, we

have also seen significant improvements in other areas, too. It is as if once you have enabled the brain's ability to learn and automatise it has a knock-on benefit for other problems, which may well prove to have their cause rooted in the same area of the brain – who knows?

The problem is that in order to do this we will need resources that we simply do not have at this present time. However, I will not let the issue rest at that. Currently, I am working hard to find research partners in universities or other organisations that want to work with us. Already we are collecting relevant data that will prove useful, but these projects are all very substantial in their own right and deserve their own dedicated research teams.

CHANGING THE WHOLE APPROACH TO LEARNING DIFFICULTIES: THE WAY FORWARD
Screening tests
At the moment, deciding how to help a child that you have just discovered has a learning difficulty can be a complete nightmare for many parents. They are likely to be bombarded with messages from all sorts of organisations, including our own, about which is the best way to go. Some tell them to try tinted lenses, others recommend prescription drugs, to go and see an educational psychologist, to see a teacher, to go on the Dore Programme, to try changing their nutrition, and so on. No one seems to be providing a holistic approach and helping them make good and appropriate choices. Families are inundated with well-meaning advice and marketing for services and programmes that have no clear benchmarking that gives any hint of which of these is the best path to take.

I feel that this situation requires drastic and urgent change. Currently, I am working with Professor Rod Nicolson on a plan to

influence researchers, associations and government bodies to start drawing up a whole series of guidelines and benchmarking standards that will help families determine the best way to identify which remedy is the most appropriate for them. I, therefore, want there to be a national screening test that will take the pain, emotion and confusion out of identifying whether or not a child has a problem that is hiding their true potential. The earlier in life the problem is identified and resolved, the happier the children's school life becomes and the more they learn. This would need to be a two-part process.

If a child displays learning or attention difficulties, then first of all it is necessary to determine if there is a physiological issue before trying to increase or change the educational support they are getting. In other words, there is no point trying to fill a bucket if it still has a hole in it – we need to repair the hole first. If there is a physiological issue, the screening test I propose will help determine the best intervention to deal with the root cause of the problem. That problem can then be tackled and, we now know, can often be corrected

Once that has been done, the second phase of screening can take place to determine what a person's educational needs are – the areas they have missed out on because of their learning difficulty. From this can be determined the best way of providing them with educational resources. Following on from a programme that corrects the ability to learn and to concentrate, many young children who are in a good school will find that the education provided is likely to be enough to help them catch up. However, if children are in their mid-teens, they may have missed out on some fundamental aspects and are no longer surrounded by those teachers with the time to help them plug vital gaps in their knowledge. These lessons, therefore, must be revisited. For

adults, the same thing will apply and they may well need one-on-one tutoring to provide the education they could not benefit from when they were in school themselves.

The technology and knowledge exists for these screening tests to be developed and used. When they are, it will help make governments aware just how prevalent the problem is. The good news for parents and teachers is that it will take away much of the emotion and doubt they have at present while providing them with a clear root map to get their child to where they could have been, had they never had a learning difficulty.

The need for benchmarking

One of the fundamental concerns I have is that, whatever treatments or programmes are made available for people to use, they must be benchmarked to an international standard. It is crucial that anything provided to people to help them with learning issues actually does help – and the degree to which they help, and which symptoms are helped is scientifically measured and reported on. It is vital that all organisations providing treatments are fully prepared to be open about the effectiveness of what they provide.

As soon as we began our research, I started asking for guidance about benchmarking, expecting that some national – if not international – institution would have dealt with this particular need. Eventually, I realised no one has taken the initiative but I am sure that with some effort we will find some very capable organisations that will do so in the near future.

I know that what we are doing in our own research programme stands up to scrutiny, but I also suspect that some other treatments do not. No one in their right mind would ever buy a car or TV set without knowing that it had been produced under proper

quality controls and conditions. So why is it that we buy resources for our children without insisting on that same degree of quality control? As an organisation, we have made it our business to have far more research supporting us than many institutions, some showing no interest at all in rigorous testing.

It pains me that many parents who have a child with learning difficulties are faced with so many confusing messages and yet are not given the crucial information to make informed decisions. As a result, they will often try a number of different treatments, each one often ending in yet more disappointment, which then discourages them from trying something else. We have often had potential users of our programme put off by the fact that everything else they have tried has ended in disappointment. Benchmarking will help stop that happening.

Attitudes

If this book has highlighted anything, it shows that we can now effectively tackle the physiological cause of many learning, attention and behavioural difficulties. Hopefully this will have a huge impact on everyone, including teachers, who will see that, once the underlying cause of learning difficulties has been dealt with, those helped start to learn much more quickly than they did before their true potential was unlocked.

Setting up a charity

When I started the programme, my initial reaction was that I should do it through a charity. This was because the driving force behind the programme was to put something back. However, when I discussed this with my advisers, I realised it was unfeasible. The ideas we were pursuing were not at that time supported by conventional wisdom or the Establishment, so the

only way forward was to set it up as a normal commercial company. This would give us the freedom to take the huge risks necessary and to spend money without being constrained.

However, as time has gone on, we have increasingly gained more and more support for our work. So the time has now come when it is appropriate to form a charity. What we have unearthed is a branch of science, which I hope will have an enormous impact on many areas. In addition, I want to have a vehicle where others worldwide will be able to share the research we do. So, I have formed a charity and called it The Dore Foundation. It has the very specific brief of masterminding the kind of research that will involve co-operation with other eminent research organisations.

The charity is being driven by some wonderful people including Peter Morley, CBE, the once head of the National Training Organization (NTO), Dr Lady Anne Redgrave, the wife of the Olympic rower Sir Steve Redgrave, and Lady Mary Nicolson, whose contribution and support have been outstanding. We already have a few projects lined up. We are going to look at how we might help reduce crime; we want to look at behavioural issues; we want to look at autism and we want to look at the development of screening tests that can be developed for use in every school. As the funding starts to flow in, these projects will be driven hard and be fully accountable, I can assure you.

One of the first major projects will be to drive for the establishment of appropriate benchmarking for all the interventions that are available – that is, all the tools, the methods, ideas and programmes available for folk with learning difficulties. This work will ensure that finally there is a worldwide benchmark that is recognised and insisted upon. When families come to choose a treatment for learning difficulties, they can look

at the research and make an informed choice about the best option for them.

Once all these visions have materialised, the world will think totally differently about people with learning difficulties. Instead of looking at these people as if something is wrong with them, they will look at them and know that there are some wonderful things hidden inside their minds: an amazing treasure trove of skills and talents just waiting to be revealed.

Chapter 17

ONE FINAL THOUGHT

My burning desire at the start was to help my daughter Susie have a normal happy life; I certainly never thought about creating an organisation. All I knew was that, if things had continued as they were, Susie was not going to live. My focus was purely and simply to enable her to have a sense of fulfilment in life. It was only in trying to resolve her problem that I realised there were so many others who faced exactly the same crisis to a greater or lesser extent every day.

It is with great relief that I can say as a father that my daughter's life has been transformed. She is a joy to be around and finally I am able to get to know the person who was locked inside of her for so many years. I remember having such an epiphany when I was travelling down to London with Susie for a conference. While waiting on the platform, to my astonishment Susie bought a copy of *Woman's Own* and proceeded to read it from cover to cover on the train. For most people, this simple act would be nothing to get excited about. However, right up until she

was in her mid-twenties, reading was something Susie would run a mile from. Having gone through the treatment, suddenly she was now reading of her own free will.

For once, I felt utterly speechless. Susie had been called 'thick', 'lazy' and 'stupid' so many times. None of those insults had ever been true. In fact, she worked twice as hard as everyone else to try to keep up with her classmates. Now, sitting beside me on the train, I had the definitive proof that my daughter was no different to anybody else. It was a beautiful moment.

Consequently, the future is now brighter for those with learning difficulties. Though we still have the hurdle to overcome of getting this paradigm shift accepted by everyone, we have started that process and the results are undeniable. So now, in the main, it is only those with vested interests that are still denying that this breakthrough is very exciting. We could forgive them before for saying this because science had not taught us what we now know. But we can't forgive them for much longer: this is not just about academic or career improvement; it concerns the very enjoyment of life itself. Such closed-mindedness is very harmful and shows no regard for the struggle millions face every day.

At the same time, hosts of others are saying that their life has been changed in a way that they could only have dreamed of before. And the more they experience it, the more the voices of those still wedded to old-fashioned theories will be silenced and the quicker governments will open their eyes to what may have monumental impact at the individual, social and economic levels. It is clear from government statistics that conventional wisdom has not led the world to strategies that have had the desired impact on reducing literacy, tackling crime and drug addiction, helping with the issues around suicide and many complex

psychiatric problems. Perhaps, with help from those research organisations with the appropriate resources, it is time to have a good look at what can be achieved just by developing the cerebellum in a natural, drug-free way.

My hope for this book is that it will go some way towards forcing the hands of many politicians and world leaders to do something with it. I personally won't be stopping until they have recognised that there is a breakthrough for learning difficulties because, until they do, this treatment will not reach everyone and further generations will suffer needlessly. Everyone reading this book will have recognised in it a description of someone they know who is underachieving as a consequence of learning or concentration issues – now we can give them hope.

TESTIMONIALS

In the following pages, I have included just a handful of testimonials I have received from children and their parents who have been on the Dore Programme. Read for yourself the effect that it has had on there lives. For every one you read here, I have a hundred more examples of positive feedback ...

BEN FEATHERSTONE (11 YEARS)

Mrs Janine Featherstone wrote:

'We will always be grateful to you all because the many improvements in all aspects of his life since going on the programme mean that Ben now has a much better life and his future looks so much more promising. Ben used to say he was going to work in kennels or a zoo because he loved animals. He now thinks he would like to be a vet! We cannot thank you enough for the help you have given to us all.'

Ben Featherstone wrote:

'I look forward to going to the Dore Centre. The people there are really nice to me and are very kind. I was glad to see that so many people have the same problems as me – I thought I was the only one. I am happier now because work is not so hard at school and I can understand things better. My memory is better, too. In my mock SATs exams, I got 2, 2, 3 in English, maths and science. After three months at Dore, I got 4, 4, 5 in my exams – that was above the national average.

'I never get car-sickness now; I am getting better at rugby, so have more friends. I now have more confidence and now I think when I leave school I will get a good job because I believe I can do my school work now.'

OLIVIA PYECROFT (13 YEARS)

Mrs Anne Pyecroft wrote:

'We watched the Trevor MacDonald programme featuring Dore together. Olivia asked if she could go there and counted down the days to her first appointment. At times, especially at the beginning, Olivia became very irritable with the demands of the exercises and I had my doubts that she would gain anything at all. However, we soon got into a routine and very soon had a positive sign that something was happening – suddenly Olivia could tell the time!

'Shortly after this, she began to form her own circle of new friends. Family friends who were not aware that she was on the programme started to comment on how she was "growing up". Her whole demeanour became more confident and her end-of-year report contained comments such as "confidence continues to improve" and "netball skills show increased improvement", etc.

'Olivia completed the programme after 12 months and she continues to improve and is now able to understand algebra and ratios.'

REBECCA DAVIES (13 YEARS)

Mrs Sue Davies wrote:

'After 21 months, we have finished the programme at the centre and I feel I have to write to give hope and encouragement to any parent starting on this course of treatment. Like almost all of the parents of the children attending the clinic, we had begun to think that we were banging our heads against a brick wall trying to get help for our daughter.

'Due to the fact that she could not express herself on paper she was treated as thick, stupid and unable to learn. The fact that no one listened to the information coming out of her mouth made the problem even harder. As a teacher, I knew there was a major problem and started looking for an answer. In the end we had to change both school and education authority to ensure that she received the help she needed. This action cost Rebecca almost two years' schooling when she was really not even holding water in her educational programme.

'The programme will not work if the child is not prepared to make the effort. The child must understand the importance of being dedicated to the exercise programme and completing them to the best of their ability. Some of the exercises that seem simple to others are extremely difficult for those with learning difficulties – did I hate it when Rebecca had to hop! But, before the first month was over, we knew that she was improving. Silly little things, but things she could not do before – tying shoelaces without having to think about it, for example.

'Her attitude in school and her work improved at a rate no one

would have thought possible. She went from a child at the end of Key Stage 1 that was barely on the line. She improved in five terms to a child that achieved above the national average, a result that would not have been possible without the programme and Rebecca's determination to improve and prove everyone wrong.

'We all know that the programme works and, without it, Rebecca would have been written off by an educational system that is unable to cope with bright, intelligent children that happen to be dyslexic. As a member of a profession that can be extremely stubborn in its approach to new ideas and its reluctance to admit that other systems work, I am convinced that this programme works and should be accepted by the educational system as a standard approach to teach children with this special educational need.

'We will keep in touch and thanks again. May you continue to have the success that you all rightly deserve.'

ALEXANDRA MOBBS (11 YEARS)

Mrs Lesley Mobbs wrote:

'Alex had problems no one could put their finger on. She was well behaved, worked hard at school and was obviously bright in so many ways, but her parents grew more and more worried about the youngster. They couldn't pinpoint what it was but just felt Alex was not achieving as much as she could have done. Alex was finally diagnosed as having attention deficit syndrome and, with the help of Dore, the 11-year-old's future is looking brighter.

'And the changes that have been seen? There are many. Because one member of staff at school knew Alex could do well, she ensured Alex was put in the top class of her year. Alex has maintained her place in that class with very high exam results. She is organised at school and home, and comes with the right equipment at the right lessons. She concentrates in class – no

more looking out of the window. If asked to tidy her room at home, she now goes and does it and is not lost for several hours. She has applied herself and gained a place at her next school in the face of stiff competition. She is reading harder books. She has become a more confident child and her self-esteem has increased. She now believes in herself and what she can do. She knows that she can do things just as well as anyone else. She is a happy child.

'Without this exercise programme, I believe that Alex would have continued to struggle unknowingly to achieve her real potential. I do not know exactly how it works, but I thank the Dore Centre for this programme and for giving Alex a chance.'